The AIMS Guide to

Induction of Labour

An AIMS Publication

Principal Author: Nadia Higson, Ph.D.
AIMS Trustee

Published by AIMS

www.aims.org.uk

publications@aims.org.uk

Tel: 0300 365 0663

© AIMS 2020

Association for Improvements in the Maternity Services

Registered Charity number 1157845

ISBN: 978-1-874413493

A catalogue record for this book is available from the British Library.

Printed in the Czech Republic by Printo

About AIMS

The Association for Improvements in the Maternity Services (AIMS) has been at the forefront of the childbirth movement since 1960. It is a volunteer-run charity and most of its work is carried out by volunteers without payment.

AIMS' day-to-day work includes providing independent support and information about maternity choices and raising awareness of current research on childbirth and related issues. AIMS actively supports parents, midwives, doctors and birth workers who recognise that, for the majority of women, birth is a normal rather than a medical event. AIMS campaigns tirelessly on many issues covered by the Human Rights legislation.

AIMS campaigns internationally, nationally and locally for better births for all, protecting human rights in childbirth and the provision of objective, evidence based information to enable informed decision making.

AIMS Mission
"We support all maternity service users to navigate the system as it exists, and campaign for a system which truly meets the needs of all."

AIMS Equality, Diversity and Inclusivity Statement

AIMS Equality, Diversity and Inclusivity Statement is available on the AIMS website at *www.aims.org.uk/general/aims-equality-diversity-and-inclusivity-statement.*

AIMS promotes equality, values diversity and challenges discrimination and with this statement we make a commitment to do so irrespective of characteristics. Freedom of expression is fundamental to AIMS and we will endeavour to publish diverse voices and wide-ranging opinions.

AIMS will work towards ensuring that all our written works will be made available in a variety of formats to meet different needs and that the language is inclusive to all.

AIMS wishes to support everyone throughout their pregnancy, ensuring that they are protected, included, celebrated and retain autonomy over their bodies.

Acknowledgements

Whilst I am the principal researcher and author for this book, like all AIMS publications it has benefitted immensely from the critical comments and suggestions of a group of AIMS volunteers. It is this approach, drawing on the knowledge and insight of both expert and lay readers, which ensures that AIMS books meet the needs of our main audience, the individual maternity service user, as well as providing valuable information to those who support them. I am grateful to all the peer reviewers for the time they have spent on this, but especially to Debbie Chippington Derrick and Jo Dagustun for their detailed input. Debbie also spent a huge amount of time going through various versions of the text with me. I am extremely grateful for her eagle eye for where more information or clearer wording was needed.

I am particularly grateful to Deborah Hughes for her expert input on diabetes and gestational diabetes and to Jessie Wise for explaining cervical ripening and the Bishop's score from a midwife's perspective.

Thanks are also due to our editor, Alison Melvin, who also typeset the manuscript, Michele Donnison at Primrose and Bee for the illustrations, Chloe Bayfield for proofreading, and our printer in the Czech Republic, Daniel Zabek.

Nadia Higson, PhD.
AIMS Trustee and Principal Author

Contents

Introduction

The AIMS Guide to Induction of Labour provides essential, evidence-based information to help you make decisions about induction of labour. It is intended to give you an understanding of:

- What is involved in an induction of labour.
- Things to consider when deciding whether it is the right option for you.
- The evidence about benefits and risks in different situations.
- The options you may have during the process.
- How to prepare if you decide to have your labour induced.

This is a reference book to be dipped into when necessary. You may only want to read about the specific reason why you are being offered an induction or to help you plan for one. We cover all methods of inducing labour, by which we mean any way of trying to start the process of labour. This includes both medical inductions, where a midwife or doctor carries out one or more procedures designed to encourage the onset of active labour, and non-medical induction including complementary therapies and self-help methods which you might use to try to bring forward the start of your labour.

This book will give you details of the available research evidence, but also make clear when there is a lack of good evidence. For an explanation of the strengths and weaknesses of different types of research evidence see AIMS Birth Information web page "Understanding Quantitative Research Evidence", *www.aims.org.uk/information/item/quantitative-research*. We also summarise the key points of the research, so if you do not want to look at the detail you can go directly to the summary. To make it easier to find, this is formatted like this, » » » **Summary.**

Interpretations of research evidence vary, and the conclusions drawn often differ depending on the views of those making them. This is why AIMS suggests that you keep asking questions to get the information that you need and then make up your own mind about what you want to do (*see "Discussing induction with doctors and midwives", p.8*).

Childbirth is usually a normal physiological process. Sometimes induction of labour or other medical interventions will be beneficial, but you have the legal right to decide not to have any intervention that is offered. There is almost always an alternative, including the option to wait and see. (*See "Informed Consent", p.1 and "BRAIN – a decision-making tool", p.7.*)

Often the reason given for recommending induction is to reduce the chances of a stillbirth. Whilst stillbirth is understandably one of the biggest fears of both parents and their doctors and midwives, the risk is usually low, and needs to be balanced against the risks of inducing labour. Induction can lead to harm to both the baby and the mother or pregnant person with no benefit for most. We have highlighted what is known about the scale of the benefits and the risks in this book. It is important to understand that where there is a benefit there may also be a risk attached, and it is for the individual to decide how they feel about the balance of risks and benefits.

Much of the research about induction of labour is necessarily quantitative (to do with numbers and measurement) rather than qualitative (descriptive). This means there is little research on how people find the experience of having labour induced. There is also a lack of research into what the long-term physical or mental consequences of induction might be for you and your baby.

It is common for induction to be offered routinely at around 40-42 weeks. It has become an expectation, not just from doctors and midwives, but also from family, friends and work colleagues, that if your labour has not begun by then that you will have this intervention. This can make it difficult to refuse it, but the choice is always yours. We hope that the information in this book will help you to decide.

Sometimes the need to induce labour is vital for the person who is pregnant and/or for their baby. In the UK, we are very lucky to have midwives and obstetricians who have the skills and equipment to intervene where needed.

Unfortunately, the AIMS Helpline frequently hears from people who feel coerced into accepting induction, often with little or no explanation of the risks and benefits from their doctor or midwife. At worst, there are threats about what might happen to their baby if they don't agree to an induction. We also hear from those who are not being listened to when they try to tell their midwife or doctor that they are worried about their baby. In either case, we hope the information and strategies suggested in this book will help you to make decisions that are right for you and your baby, and to have those decision supported.

We know that some people have found induction of labour difficult and stressful, but for others it can be a positive experience. If you have decided that induction is right for you there will usually be options for how and where the process is carried out, and what kind of support will be available to you. This can make a big difference to the experience – so don't hesitate to ask for what you would prefer. You will find information on this in the section *"Planning for an induction of labour", p.135*.

If you are interested in the 'politics' of why there has been a huge increase in the rates of induction in recent years, there is more information in the AIMS Journal 2019, Vol 31, no 1, *To Induce or not to Induce – at least ask the question? www.aims.org.uk/journal/index/31/1*. It is a good companion to this book.

How to get the best out of this book – an explanation of its structure
Chapter I explains your rights and how to make the decision about induction of labour which is best for you. It gives information about consent, evidence-based information and how to get the information you need from your midwife or doctor.

Chapter 2 discusses the reasons you might be offered an induction of labour. The structure of this section gives you details of the research evidence and a list of 'things to consider' when making your decision. There is a lot of research for most of the situations, so we have included summaries at the end of each section. The research evidence is highlighted like this, ◈ ◈ ◈ **Research Evidence,** the summaries like this, » » » **Summary** and considerations like this, ∼∼∼ Things to consider.

Chapter 3 explains how spontaneous labour begins, provides information about non-medical and medical induction methods and the evidence on the benefits and risks of each method. There is a very helpful chart on page 140 highlighting the decision points at each stage of the induction process. This chapter also covers things that may help an induction to work, what having a medical induction might mean for your labour, and suggestions on planning for one.

There is a Glossary on page 139, and online at *www.aims.org.uk/general/glossary,* which explains the medical and technical terms used throughout the book. These are indicated by **bold** text.

Useful resources can be found on *www.aims.org.uk/general/induction.*

Language

AIMS understands that there is a huge diversity of people who use the maternity services. AIMS seeks to support all users, so we have tried to make the language in this book inclusive. Much of the time we use 'you' – directed at the reader who will usually be the maternity service user. We use the terms mothers or women when discussing research or guidelines in line with what the authors have used. Elsewhere we have used a mix of women, mothers, people, or pregnant women and people to reflect the fact that some of those who give birth do not identify as women.

Get support from the AIMS Helpline

The book is full of information but if you have specific questions or want to discuss anything about induction, or anything relating to labour, birth or the maternity services please contact: *helpline@aims.org.uk* or +44 (0) 300 3650663. This phone number will connect you to an AIMS volunteer when possible; if no one is available please leave us a message, or email us, and someone will get back to you.

About the principal author

Dr Nadia Higson has a B.A. in Natural Sciences from the University of Cambridge, and a Ph.D. in Molecular Biology. She has a Diploma in Antenatal Education and has been facilitating antenatal courses for the NCT since 2000.

She is a user representative on the Maternity Voices Partnership at her local NHS Hospital Trust, a Trustee of AIMS and volunteers on the AIMS Helpline, providing evidence-based information and support to maternity service users and those who support them.

Chapter 1

Making the right decision for you

Everyone has a legal right to make their own decisions about the healthcare they receive, and that includes care before, during and after birth. They also have the right to decline any medical tests or treatments which are offered to them. The NICE Guidelines on Inducing Labour (NICE 2008) says:

> "Treatment and care should take into account women's individual needs and preferences. Women who are having or being offered induction of labour should have the opportunity to make informed decisions about their care and treatment, in partnership with their healthcare professionals…

> "Good communication between healthcare professionals and women is essential. It should be supported by evidence-based written information tailored to the needs of the individual woman."

Informed consent

Doctors and midwives have a legal duty to ensure that a person has given 'informed consent' before they carry out any procedure, however routine or minor. This means that they should provide evidence-based information about the proposed treatment and any possible alternatives, including the option of simply waiting to see how things develop, and about any significant risks that there might be with each option. This is confirmed by the Royal College of Obstetricians and Gynaecologists' guidance for doctors on obtaining consent (RCOG 2015b), which says:

> "Before seeking a woman's consent for a test, treatment, intervention or operation, you should ensure that she is fully informed, understands the nature of the condition for which it is being proposed, its prognosis, likely consequences and the risks of receiving no treatment, as well as any reasonable or accepted alternative treatments."

The information should be objective, and presented without any attempt to bully, threaten or otherwise unduly influence someone into agreeing to the midwife or doctor's recommended course of action.

The only exceptions to this are if a person does not have the mental capacity to consent, or in an emergency where they are physically unable to consent. Otherwise, a midwife or doctor who carries out any procedure without having gained informed consent is breaking the law.

Midwives and doctors are there to advise and support you. It is reasonable for a doctor or midwife to make a recommendation, but they should explain their reasons for doing so. It's then up to you to decide how you feel about the information they have given you and what you want to do about it. The principle of informed consent also has to allow for 'informed withholding of consent.' If you decide against following your doctor or midwife's recommendation, they should support you in your decision.

You may be told that induction or another medical procedure is hospital policy or recommended by guidelines. It's important to realise that hospital policies or guidelines are there to tell staff what treatment to offer but it's up to you whether to accept it. Guidelines are not rules that you have to follow and must not be used to deny you the right to make your own decisions.

Ideally recommendation made by doctors and midwives will be based on up-to-date, good quality research evidence, but sadly this is always not the case.

If you do not feel your midwife or doctor has given you enough information to enable you to decide, then you have every right to ask them for what you need. You also have the right to take whatever time you need to consider your options and should not be pressed to make a decision on the spot.

If your midwife or doctor has not followed these principles, then legally you have not given your informed consent for them to carry out the procedure and they could potentially be sued for negligence.

For more information on the principle of consent and your legal rights, see the factsheet "Consenting to Treatment" produced by the charity Birth Rights at *https://birthrights.org.uk/wp-content/uploads/2019/03/Consenting-to-treatment-2019.pdf*.

About NICE and other guidelines

Throughout this book you will find references to guidelines published by the National Institute for Health and Care Excellence (NICE), especially the NICE guideline "Inducing Labour" (NICE 2008). These guidelines are produced by Guideline Development Groups (**GDG**) and contain recommendations which are intended to be based on the best available evidence. In some cases where there is insufficient evidence, they may just reflect what the GDG agreed was 'good practice'. They may also make recommendations for further research.

Hospitals are not obliged to follow NICE recommendations but should do so in deciding on their routine practice. Recommendations are not rules that you have to follow, they are about the care that you should be offered.

The guideline on induction covers various situations in which the GDG thought induction should and should not be offered. These guidelines have been in place 2008, so it's possible some of the recommendations outlined below will be revised in the next version.

You can find an explanation of the role of NICE here *www.nice.org. uk/about/what-we-do* and an outline of how they develop guidelines here *www.nice.org.uk/about/what-we-do/our-programmes/nice-guidance/nice-guidelines/ how-we-develop-nice-guidelines.*

Other guidelines are published by the professional bodies which regulate midwives and doctors, called the Royal College of Midwives (RCM) and the Royal College of Obstetricians and Gynaecologists (RCOG). You can find many examples of maternity guidelines on their websites *www.rcm.org.uk* (Blue Top Guidance) and *www.rcog.org.uk* (Green Top Guidance). These are based on published research and provide recommendations about appropriate treatment in different circumstances, but they do not dictate a single solution. The responsibility for your care still lies with your midwife or doctor and should always take account of your individual wishes and needs.

About evidence-based information

At AIMS we always do our best to make sure that the information we give is evidence-based. Unfortunately, evidence is often not clear-cut or may be lacking altogether, and sometimes the research that has been done is of poor quality. In this book we have tried to explain what evidence there is about induction in different situations, and the limits of that evidence.

In any kind of research, grouping people together according to one characteristic, such as age, BMI or the fact that they conceived through IVF, often ignores the fact that there could be important differences between the individuals in a group. For example, pregnancy and birth outcomes might be very different for someone over 40 who has a healthy lifestyle, is completely well and has had a straightforward pregnancy, compared to someone who has existing health problems, or who smokes or drinks heavily, yet recommendations may be made based purely on their age.

In thinking about what research evidence can tell us, it's important to keep these limitations in mind.

In this book we generally quote **absolute risks**, as these are more helpful than **relative risks** for people who are trying to make decisions. How people feel about risk is a matter of personal attitudes, values and circumstances. One person might consider a risk of an extra one in 100 to be too small to worry about, but another might decide one in 1000 is too great a risk to take. Midwives and doctors will often focus on one specific risk and ignore other things which may be very important to you.

If you are interested in learning more about this, see the AIMS Birth Information web page "Understanding Quantitative Research Evidence", *www.aims.org.uk/information/item/quantitative-research.*

Making decisions about induction

The most common reason given for induction of labour is to try to reduce the risk of a baby being stillborn. Less often, there may be a cause for concern about the mother or pregnant person's health if the pregnancy were to continue. In some circumstances we have good evidence that an **early birth**, by induction or **planned caesarean**, is likely to be beneficial or even life-saving. However, the quality of the evidence for induction in other situations varies a lot, and in many cases is much more limited and contradictory than the information that is often given to parents would suggest.

In recent years the number of labours being induced has risen dramatically from just over 20% in 2007– 08 to almost 33% in 2017–18 (National Maternity Statistics for 2017–18) and it is questionable how many of these were justified.

Sometimes there is evidence to support the belief that a policy of induction will reduce the number of stillbirths, but because the risk is low a very large number of labours would need to be induced to avoid one stillbirth. The difficulty is that there is often no way of telling the few babies who would benefit from an earlier birth from the vast majority who can safely wait for labour to begin. In other cases evidence for the benefit of induction is not at all clear-cut, and sometimes it is virtually non-existent.

You may want to consider which view you feel more comfortable with: "Induction might help, so why not do it just in case?" or "There's no evidence that induction does any good, so why do it?" We discuss the evidence concerning induction for various common reasons in *Chapter 2, Reasons for Induction of Labour, p.16*.

It is worth remembering that induction whether medical or non-medical is *always* an attempt to persuade your body to go into labour before your baby is ready to be born. This may be justified if there is a risk to your or your baby's health, but any kind of intervention in the natural process is likely to have some consequences. Also, no method of induction is guaranteed to work, so it's worth considering what your options would be if your labour does not start.

As described below, medical induction methods can have both short-term and potentially long-term consequences for the physical and emotional health of mothers and babies. A recent review of stillbirth rates in the Netherlands (Seijmonsbergen-Schermers 2019) argues that "Induction of labor should only be offered to individual women if there is a medical necessity... we argue that a small absolute increase in risk on its own, without any other medical risks or complications during pregnancy, does not justify a policy of routinely offering induction of labor without strong evidence of the benefits of that policy."

For any decision, it can be helpful to use the 'BRAIN' questions:

BRAIN: A decision-making tool

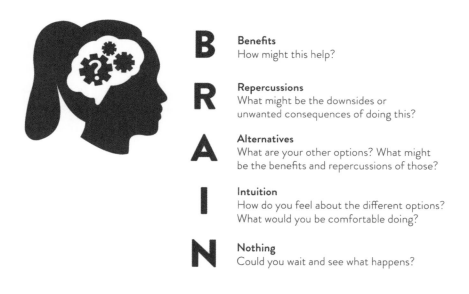

B Benefits
How might this help?

R Repercussions
What might be the downsides or
unwanted consequences of doing this?

A Alternatives
What are your other options? What might
be the benefits and repercussions of those?

I Intuition
How do you feel about the different options?
What would you be comfortable doing?

N Nothing
Could you wait and see what happens?

In the case of an offer of medical induction, other alternatives could be to wait a while longer for labour to start (**expectant management** – the 'do nothing' option), to try non-medical methods (*see "Non-medical methods of induction" p.106*) or to plan a **caesarean**.

There will almost always be a trade-off between the benefits and repercussions of each alternative, and how you view this will depend on your own attitudes, needs and priorities.

It is for you to say what risks are and are not acceptable to you. No one has the right to decide that for you. If you prefer to wait for spontaneous labour, you can also decide whether to accept additional monitoring of your and your baby's well-being in the meantime.

For further discussion of making decisions see the AIMS Birth Information web page *www.aims.org.uk/information/item/making-decisions*.

Discussing induction with doctors and midwives

It is the responsibility of your midwife or doctor to give you the answers you need to enable you to make an informed decision, so don't be put off if they seem to brush your questions aside or give you unsatisfactory answers. It may help to keep repeating your question until they answer it to your satisfaction. You may find it helpful to:

- Write a note of the questions that you want them to answer.
- Take someone else with you, to give you support and to remind you about what you wanted to ask. That could be your partner, another family member or friend, or a doula (trained birth supporter).
- Ask for time to write down the answers, or you may want to ask whether you can record the conversation for your reference.
- Ask for references to the research which supports their recommendation, if you want to be able to look it up for yourself.

The sort of questions you might want to ask your midwife or doctor include:

- Do you have any concern about my or my baby's well-being right now?
- Why do you think that my baby needs to be born at x weeks? What is the evidence on which you are basing that recommendation?
- If this is hospital policy, what research evidence is that based on?
- How do you think induction at x weeks will benefit me and my baby?

- What are the potential risks for me and my baby of having labour induced at this stage of pregnancy and how great are those risks? Asking them to tell you the absolute risk e.g. "this might happen in x out of every 1000 cases" can make it easier to weigh things up rather than if they just say that something 'increases' or 'doubles' the risk without telling you how big that risk is.
- What impact might having an induced labour have on me and my baby in the long term?
- What percentage of inductions at this stage of pregnancy are successful? How likely is it to be successful in my case?
- How long might it take from the start of the induction process until I am in active labour?
- What would my options be if the induction is unsuccessful?
- What are the potential risks if I choose to wait to go into labour and how great are those risks in actual numbers?
- What are the potential risks if I choose to have a planned **caesarean** and how great are those risks in actual numbers?
- How would you monitor my baby's well-being if I decided to wait a while longer?

You might also want to ask your midwife or doctor about when, where and how the induction could be carried out (as practice varies between hospitals), whether there is a choice of methods, and what pain relief and support you would be offered at different points in the process. There is a list of these and other things that you might want to ask or think about in *"Planning for an induction of labour", p.135.*

Unless your midwife or doctor are saying that there is an immediate need for your baby to be born, you do not have to decide then and there. It may be helpful to say something like, "Thank you for the information. I will think it over and let you know in a couple of days what I have decided to do." This can also be a way of politely closing a discussion you are finding unhelpful, for example, if you feel that someone is trying to pressurise you into agreeing to something that you are not sure about.

If you are unsure about any recommendation, you have the right to ask for a second opinion. Second opinions should be from a consultant obstetrician rather than a less senior doctor. This also applies to any decision that you might be making during a medical induction.

You may be told that you need to book the date for an induction because the slots get booked up. It's obviously easier for the hospital if they know how many people are coming in for induction on a given day, but they would be failing in their duty of care if they refused you an induction you needed simply because you had not made an appointment for it in advance. Some people will choose to allow the hospital to make a booking, and others may find that they have been booked in for an induction which they have not agreed to and do not want. Remember that you are not obliged to keep an appointment just because someone else has made it.

Do I have to be induced?

Mothers and pregnant people are often told by their midwives or doctors that they will 'have' to be induced by a certain date or will only be 'allowed' to wait till a certain number of weeks of pregnancy before having their labour induced. This is incorrect. It is *always* your choice whether to accept advice to have your labour medically induced, and at what point in your pregnancy to do that. No one can force you to go to hospital and no one can legally carry out any medical procedure if you have not given your informed consent to it.

Some people, if they agree that an **early birth** is appropriate, will prefer an induction of labour in the hope of then having a vaginal birth, and others will prefer a planned caesarean. Your consultant should give you full information on the risks and benefits of both these options, as well as the option of waiting for your labour to start.

You can find out more about the comparative risks of vaginal and caesarean birth in the NICE caesarean guideline (NICE 2011 *www.nice.org. uk/guidance/cg132/ifp/chapter/Risks-of-caesarean-section*) and in this article on the AIMS website *www.aims.org.uk/information/item/caesarean*.

Do I have the right to choose an induction?

You may have a reason to want your baby to be born at a particular time. This might be so your partner can be with you, or family will be available to help after the birth. It could also be because you are struggling to cope with the effects of pregnancy or are worried about your baby.

Although anyone has the right to decline a treatment or procedure, they do not have a right to receive it. The NICE guidelines (NICE 2008) say "Induction of labour should not routinely be offered on maternal request alone. However, under exceptional circumstances (for example, if the woman's partner is soon to be posted abroad with the armed forces), induction may be considered at or after 40 weeks." The full version of the guideline has a stronger wording: "The **GDG** considered the dialogue between the woman and the clinician in making any decision about management to be important, and *a case-by-case approach, taking into account the woman's clinical and personal circumstances, is appropriate*" (our italics).

This means that if you have a strong personal reason for requesting an induction your doctor should be prepared to discuss it. This applies even if they see no medical need for it. If you want to do this you will need to think through your reasons and make sure you can explain them firmly and clearly. If your doctor is unwilling to induce labour at your request, you can try changing to a different consultant or even a different hospital that has a more flexible policy.

If you want an induction because you are concerned about your baby's well-being but are being told by your doctor or midwife that they do not consider induction necessary, you have the right to ask for a second opinion.

When is induction NOT recommended?

The NICE **GDG** listed the following situations where they believed induction should not be offered (NICE 2008).

Breech babies

The GDG said that induction "is not generally recommended" if the baby is lying bottom-down (breech) rather than head down. However, it can be offered if there are concerns about leaving the pregnancy to continue, if attempts to turn the baby have failed or been declined by the mother, and if the mother does not want a caesarean.

In fact, there seems to be no good research evidence to show whether induction when the baby is breech carries any greater risks than a spontaneous labour.

Babies with severe growth problems

This refers to babies who have very poor growth *and* other worrying signs such as poor blood flow in their umbilical cord.

The GDG said that "if there is severe **fetal growth restriction** with confirmed **fetal compromise** induction of labour is not recommended." This means babies which are growing poorly and also showing signs of distress should not be subjected to the extra stress of an induced labour. However, there seems to be almost no research on the subject.

They did not comment on the situation for babies who seem to be small, but where tests of well-being have given no cause for concern.

History of fast labours

If your previous labours have been very quick, midwives or doctors will sometimes recommend induction. These very fast 'precipitate' labours (under three hours from the first contractions to birth) occur in about 2% of spontaneous labours.

If you have had a fast labour previously you might decide to request an induction to avoid the chance that you might give birth before you can get to your chosen birthplace. Alternatively, you might want to consider a homebirth (if there is no reason to birth in hospital) to avoid any worries about getting to your birthplace in time.

The **GDG** found no evidence to show that induction helped to avoid precipitate labour, and therefore concluded that it should not be offered routinely.

Suspected large baby

If there is no other cause for concern, the GDG said, "induction of labour should not be carried out simply because a healthcare professional suspects a baby is large for gestational age (**macrosomic**)".

There has been some further research on this subject since these guidelines were produced. For a discussion of this evidence see *"Induction for predicted high birthweight", p.52.*

Deciding about induction before 39 weeks

If you are recommended to have an induction at or before 39 weeks of pregnancy, you may want to consider the health problems and other consequences that can arise for a baby who is born early. The balance of risks and benefits for an induction before full term (40 weeks) will depend on how far advanced your pregnancy is as well as on the reasons why the induction is being recommended.

Premature babies (birth before 37 weeks)

The effects of **premature** birth tend to be more serious the earlier the birth occurs. Depending how early they are born, a premature baby will probably spend some time in a hospital special care unit or, if very premature or unwell, in a neonatal intensive care unit.

A premature baby has a greater risk of breathing problems because their lungs are not yet fully developed. This may mean that they need to be given extra oxygen through a mask or tube, or in more severe cases to be on a ventilator. For most babies this has no lasting effect but, rarely, it can lead to longer term breathing problems or developmental disabilities (ACOG 2013). If the birth is going to be premature you may be given a course of corticosteroids to help prepare your baby's lungs.

Premature babies are more likely to have health problems and are at greater risk of infections, both because they have underdeveloped immune systems and because they are having a lot of tests and treatments. Babies born before about 32–34 weeks will often not be able to suckle from the breast at first, and even once they are able to do this, it can take some weeks to establish breastfeeding.

Early term birth (37–39 weeks)

Often midwives and doctors will talk as though once a pregnancy reaches 37 weeks there is no issue with the baby being born early. However, there is growing evidence that key developments occur between 37 and 39 weeks of pregnancy and that **early term** babies (born between 37 and 39 weeks) are more likely to experience health problems including breathing difficulties than those born after 39 weeks. (ACOG 2013) It is for this reason that NICE recommends that planned **caesareans** "should not routinely be carried out before 39 weeks". (NICE 2011).

Am I more likely to need a caesarean?

One of the main concerns about offering induction is that it might increase the number of caesareans, either because the induction puts a baby under more stress, or because the induction fails to progress to the birth of the baby within a reasonable time.

The research evidence about the impact of induction on caesarean rates is contradictory and has been much debated by experts. In formal **randomised controlled trials** it looks as though induction does not significantly increase the chances of having a caesarean, but **population studies** suggest that in real life it's likely that it does.

For more about the research evidence, see the AIMS Birth Information web page "Am I more likely to need a caesarean if my labour is induced?", *www.aims.org.uk/information/item/induction-and-caesareans*.

Chapter 2

Reasons for induction of labour

When might induction be suggested?

There are many circumstances when doctors or midwives may recommend that your labour is induced. In this chapter we will review some of the most common ones, looking at the evidence behind such a recommendation and what that evidence can or can't tell us about the risks, benefits and repercussions of induction in each situation.

At the end of each 'reason' we offer a list of 'things to consider' when making your decision. Many of these are to do with your attitude to the trade-off of risks and benefits, or your knowledge of your body, your pregnancy or your family history. In some cases there are medical points that you may want to check with your midwife or doctor.

The following quote from a group of expert doctors is food for thought; it is in the introduction to "A Guide to Effective Care in Pregnancy & Childbirth" (Enkin 2000):

> "We worked from two basic principles: first, that the only
> justification for practices that restrict a woman's autonomy, her
> freedom of choice, and her access to her baby, would be clear
> evidence that these restrictive practices do more good than harm;

and second, that any interference with the natural process of pregnancy and childbirth should also be shown to do more good than harm. We believe that the onus of proof rests on those who advocate any intervention with either of these principles."

In some cases there will be good evidence that induction is likely to reduce the chance of harm to you and/or your baby. In other situations, there may be little or no evidence to tell us whether it is generally better if the labour is induced or not. Often the reasoning seems to be that in circumstances where there appears to be a possible risk of harm to the baby it's advisable to get them born early before any harm can happen. It could, however, be equally well argued that if these babies are at greater than average risk from the stress of labour, the last thing they need is the even higher stress that might be caused by an induction. In the absence of evidence, either view could be correct.

Length of pregnancy

It is very common to be told that there is an increased risk of stillbirth in pregnancies that last longer than 42 weeks and so labour needs to be induced before this. In fact, the interpretation of the evidence on this issue is subject to much dispute between experts.

What studies do show is that even if there is an increase in stillbirth rates beyond 42 weeks it remains rare – probably about two in 1000 **ongoing pregnancies**, compared with one to one-and-a-half in 1000 pregnancies which are ongoing at 40 weeks. Some evidence suggests that in the absence of known risk factors there is no increase in risk for mothers who wait beyond 42 weeks to give birth (Chippington Derrick & Higson, 2019). This is discussed in more detail below.

It's interesting to look at the wording that is used about this in the NICE guidelines on inducing labour (NICE 2008). These recommend that:

- Women with uncomplicated pregnancies should be given every opportunity to go into spontaneous labour.
- Women with uncomplicated pregnancies should usually be offered induction of labour between 41+0 and 42+0 weeks to avoid the risks of prolonged pregnancy. The exact timing should take into account the woman's preferences and local circumstances.
- If a woman chooses not to have induction of labour, her decision should be respected. Healthcare professionals should discuss the woman's care with her from then on.
- From 42 weeks, women who decline induction of labour should be offered increased antenatal monitoring consisting of at least twice-weekly cardiotocography and ultrasound estimation of maximum amniotic pool depth. [This means checking the baby's heartbeat and the volume of fluid surrounding them.]

This makes it absolutely clear that it is your decision whether to accept induction, and the timing of it if you do. You have the right to wait up to or even beyond 42 weeks if you wish, and your decision must be supported.

In practice, hospital policies vary (which is by itself an indication that there is no definite 'right answer') but they usually recommend induction somewhere between 41 and 42 weeks. In some circumstances, hospitals may recommend an earlier date. *(See "Your age", p.45 and "IVF pregnancy", p.92.)*

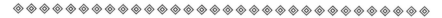

Research Evidence

The main evidence for an increase in stillbirth rates in late pregnancy comes from studies looking at the outcomes for a large population. These studies suggest that there is an increase in stillbirths in the later weeks of pregnancy, but it is a very small increase.

A review which combined data from a number of these **population studies** (Muglu 2019) found a small increase in the risk of stillbirth beyond 40 weeks. This estimated that there was one additional stillbirth for every 1,449 pregnancies which lasted to 41 weeks compared with 40 weeks and one additional stillbirth for every 604 pregnancies which lasted to 42 weeks compared with 41 weeks.

However, a population study from the UK (Cotzias 1999) which was not included in the review reported that though the risk was at its lowest at 40 weeks and rose slightly after that, beyond 42 weeks it was no higher than it was at 37-38 weeks. This corresponded to one additional stillbirth for every 1,500 mothers whose pregnancies continued to 43 weeks, compared to the rate for mothers who birthed or were still pregnant after 40 weeks. This is referred to as the number of **ongoing pregnancies**.

Stillbirths per 1000 ongoing singleton pregnancies by week of pregnancy

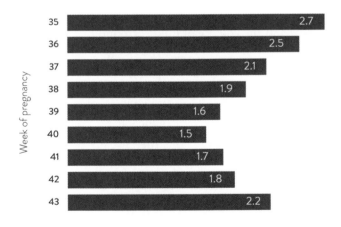

Source: Cotzias et al 1999

Another study from Norway, (Morken, 2014) looked at **perinatal deaths**, defined as stillbirths plus deaths in the first week of life. It found about two perinatal deaths per 1000 births at 42 weeks or more, compared to 1.3/1000 births at 40 weeks (so that's one additional perinatal death per 1,500 births). However, this study also suggested that the main problem may not be a longer pregnancy as such, but a longer pregnancy when the baby is not growing well. The number of deaths amongst these babies, called Small for Gestational Age (**SGA**) babies in the graph below, was greater at all weeks of pregnancy, and increased much more sharply beyond 40 weeks, than for babies who had normal growth (Non-SGA babies). For more about SGA babies see *"Induction for suspected poor growth", p.76.*

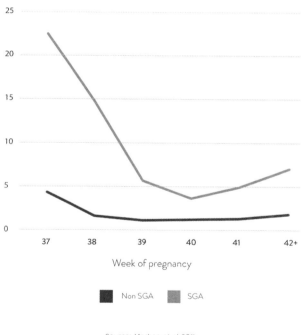

Perinatal deaths per 1000 births by week of pregnancy

Week of pregnancy

■ Non SGA   ■ SGA

Source: Morken et al 2014

Further evidence comes from a series of reports from the UK's confidential enquiries into perinatal deaths (*www.npeu.ox.ac.uk/mbrrace-uk/reports/perinatal-mortality-surveillance*). These provide data for the whole of the UK on numbers of stillbirths and **neonatal deaths** by length of pregnancy and include data on around 20,000 people each year whose pregnancies have continued to week 42 or beyond. These statistics effectively give us a recent UK based population study, which enables us to compare the outcomes of longer pregnancies with those where birth took place between 37 and 42 weeks. Over the last four years for which we have data, analysis shows that the rate of stillbirths/1000 ongoing pregnancies has generally been *lower* (or in 2014 the same) for mothers who birthed at 42 weeks or beyond than it was for all those who birthed at 37-41 weeks (Chippington Derrick & Higson 2019).

Stillbirths per 1000 ongoing pregnancies before and after 42 weeks

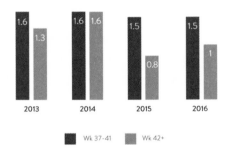

The reports also provide figures for the number of **neonatal deaths** per 1000 live births. These have consistently been lower over the last four years for babies born at or after 42 weeks than for those born between 37 and 41 weeks.

Neonatal deaths/1000 live births before and after 42 weeks

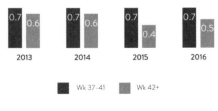

Source: MBRRACE reports 2013-2016

21

It is likely that most of those who had known medical risk factors will either have laboured spontaneously or accepted induction before 42 weeks. This data strongly suggests that in the UK in recent years people who have continued their pregnancy beyond 42 weeks have not encountered an increased risk of stillbirth or **neonatal death**.

All the evidence discussed in this section, from **meta-analyses**, **population studies** and the MBRRACE data, suggests that it is rare for an otherwise healthy baby to die even if the pregnancy goes beyond 42 weeks, and that the increase in risk beyond 42 weeks, if it exists, is small. This is in contrast to the alarmist way in which the 'risk' of longer pregnancy is often presented.

How long a pregnancy is 'too long'?

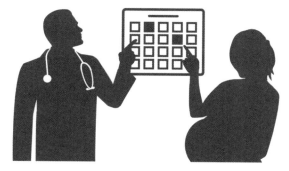

One concern about inducing labour on the grounds of the length of pregnancy is that if the estimated birth date is wrong, the baby might be born early and not be fully prepared for life outside the womb *(see "Early Term birth", p.14)*. It is very important to consider how accurate a predicted due date is.

Also, the concept of being 'overdue' implies that all babies are 'due' after the same length of pregnancy. In fact, there is plenty of evidence that there is variation in this, and that factors like both parents' genes, your ethnic heritage and your menstrual cycle can make a big difference to what would be the right length of pregnancy for your baby. It seems that some babies are genetically programmed to have longer than average pregnancies, and some to have shorter ones.

There is growing evidence that labour normally starts when the baby sends chemical signals to say that they are ready to be born *(see "Spontaneous Labour", p.104)*. Therefore, it's possible that if your labour hasn't started, this is because your baby is one who needs a bit longer to develop in the womb.

For more about these important issues see the AIMS Birth Information web page "How accurate is my due date?", *www.aims.org.uk/information/item/due-date*.

Do placentas start to fail as they age?

It is extremely common to be told that you will need to be induced if you are not in labour by 42 weeks because the placenta starts to 'fail' in late pregnancy. There is no evidence that this happens as a matter of course, or that it is responsible for late stillbirths. In fact, if it was the case it would make things easier because it might then be possible to detect which placentas were failing and induce labour only for those babies, rather than all those not yet born at 42 weeks.

If a placenta was no longer doing an efficient job of transferring nutrients to a baby this could be expected to result in the baby's growth slowing down. In contrast, one of the concerns with a long pregnancy is that the baby may grow too large, so it seems very unlikely to be the case that placentas regularly stop working properly after a certain point.

Placentas will undergo changes over time (Maiti 2017), but most placentas from longer pregnancies show no evidence of major structural abnormalities, and "There is, in fact, no logical reason for believing that the placenta, which is a fetal organ, should age while the other fetal organs do not." (Fox 1997).

Does induction by 42 weeks reduce the risk?

To answer this question there would need to be an impractically large study to be certain whether induction makes a difference to such a rare outcome as **stillbirth** or **perinatal** death. "Estimates are that a definitive study would require randomization of between 16,000 and 30,000 pregnancies. At present no such studies exist, and they will presumably never be performed." (Mandruzzato, 2010), so we are reliant on **meta-analysis** reviews. What makes it hard to interpret the findings of these is that different reviews have reached different conclusions depending on which of the many studies they chose to include.

The most recent, and largest meta-analysis (Middleton, 2018), still only included 12,000 women – so fewer than the number Mandruzzato thinks are needed for a definitive study. It also included a high proportion (13/30) of studies dating from before 1990 when maternity care may have been very different from now.

This review concluded that if 426 women had an induction before 42 weeks of pregnancy that would avoid one stillbirth. It found that fewer **caesareans**, but more **assisted births**, were required with induction compared with waiting for spontaneous labour. For more on the evidence around induction and caesareans see the AIMS Birth Information web page "Might I need a caesarean if my labour is induced?", *www.aims.org.uk/information/item/induction-and-caesareans.*

It's worth noting that the authors of the review found no difference in any of the outcomes measured whether the induction took place before or after 41 weeks of pregnancy, except that assisted births were more common with induction before 41 weeks. This review therefore does not provide evidence to support induction before 41 weeks, if the only reason is avoiding prolonged pregnancy.

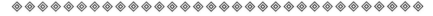

Research Evidence

Other reviews that included different sets of studies reached different conclusions. Two (Wennerholm, 2009, Sanchez-Ramos 2003) which looked only at studies of induction after 41 weeks both found that there was no **statistically significant** difference in **perinatal** deaths between the induction and **expectant management** groups. However, the total numbers in these studies are much too low to reliably detect a difference in such a rare outcome.

Another review (Mandruzzato, 2010) which looked only at trials published since 1990 found that, once babies with genetic defects or who had been growing poorly in the womb were excluded from the figures, none of the individual trials showed a significant difference in perinatal deaths.

Summary

» It is rare for an otherwise healthy baby to die even if the pregnancy goes beyond 42 weeks, and the increase in risk beyond 42 weeks, if it exists, is small.

» Although it is often raised as a concern, there is no direct evidence that placentas routinely stop working beyond 42 weeks. If a placenta was 'failing' this would probably show up in the baby's growth slowing or other signs of distress.

» There is a natural variation in the length of pregnancy, which is strongly influenced by genetics. If either parent has a family history of longer pregnancies it may be that their baby needs a bit longer to be fully prepared for life outside the womb.

» The evidence for whether induction before 42 weeks reduces the risk of stillbirth or **neonatal deaths** is contradictory. No study has been done (or probably will be done) that would be large enough to give a clear answer, and whether a **meta-analysis** finds evidence of a benefit seems to depend entirely on which studies the authors choose to include.

» Even if we accept the findings of the largest meta-analysis (Middleton 2018), it would be necessary to induce several hundred labours to avoid one baby dying, and all those other mothers and babies will have been exposed to the stress and risks of induction (see Chapter 3).

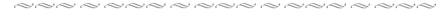

Things to consider

- Are there reasons to expect your pregnancy to be longer (or shorter) than average, for example your family history or your menstrual cycle?
- Do you have reason to question the accuracy of the estimated birth date in your notes?
- How do you feel about the risk of stillbirth if your pregnancy lasted beyond 42 weeks?
- How do you feel about the possible risks of a medical induction and the possibility of needing an unplanned **caesarean** if it fails? (*See Chapter 3*)
- Are you happy to wait a bit longer for your labour to begin? If so, do you want to accept any regular monitoring of your baby's well-being?

If your waters break before labour

Induction may be suggested if your waters break before your labour contractions have started. If this happens after 37 weeks of pregnancy it is referred to as Prelabour Rupture of the Membranes (PROM), and before 37 weeks as Preterm Prelabour Rupture of the Membranes (Pre-PROM or PPROM).

Contrary to the impression given by TV dramas, waters breaking isn't usually the first sign that labour is starting. PROM is thought to happen in about eight out of every 100 pregnancies, and Pre-PROM in about three out of every 100. For the other 90% or so of pregnant women and people, the waters will break at some point after contractions have started, and this could be at any time during the labour, though most often only once the contractions have become strong and regular (active labour). Occasionally babies are even born with the membranes which surround the waters still intact.

The concern about PROM and Pre-PROM is that once the membranes that surround the waters have broken, there is no longer a barrier to bacteria moving up and potentially causing an infection in the womb and/or affecting the baby.

There is some evidence (Seaward 1997, 1998) that the risk of infection in mother and baby increases slightly with the length of time between PROM and the start of active labour, but there are other factors, such as the number of vaginal examinations carried out, which have more impact *(see "What affects the risk of infection in the womb after PROM?", p.31, and "What affects the risk of infection for babies after PROM?", p.32).*

The guidelines for PROM and Pre-PROM are different, so we consider them separately.

Fore-waters or hind-waters?

Towards the end of pregnancy, the baby's head tends to divide the amniotic fluid inside the womb into two areas, known as the fore-waters, at the bottom of the womb, in front of the baby's head and the hind-waters, up behind the baby's head.

The waters breaking means that a small gap has opened in the amniotic membranes which contain the fluid inside the womb, allowing the fluid to leak out. If this happens in the membranes in front of the baby's head the fore-waters sometimes gush out with a distinct feeling of something popping, but sometimes it is more of a trickle. After the fore-waters have gone, fluid from the hind-waters may continue to trickle down. This isn't a problem as a baby continuously produces more fluid – the womb does not run dry.

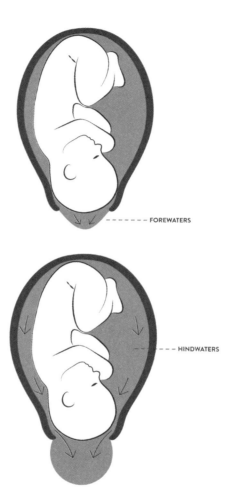

It's also possible for a small opening to develop in the membranes somewhere higher up in the womb, letting the hind-waters out. Usually this results in a trickle rather than a gush. This may continue or the membranes may re-seal themselves after a few hours or days.

The research that has been done on risks of infection after PROM does not distinguish between fore-water and hind-water leaks. It seems plausible that the risk with a hind-water leak will be lower because of the time it would take for bacteria to travel in any number all the way up from the vagina to the place where the leak occurred and by that time, the leak may have re-sealed itself.

If you are not sure whether your waters have broken you can try collecting some of the fluid on a maternity pad. It will look and smell different from urine, and there are some products on the market which enable you to test the fluid yourself. Alternatively you can ask your midwife to test the fluid for you.

Prelabour Rupture of Membranes (PROM)

The NICE Guideline on Induction (NICE 2008) made the following recommendations:

- Women with prelabour rupture of membranes at term (at or over 37 weeks) should be offered a choice of induction of labour with vaginal PGE2* or expectant management.
- Induction of labour is appropriate approximately 24 hours after prelabour rupture of the membranes at term.

*PGE2 is a form of **prostaglandin**. For more about this see *"Induction with Prostaglandin", p.113.*

The same recommendation for induction after 24 hours was repeated in the guideline on Intrapartum Care (NICE 2014, updated 2017).

Note that both sets of guidelines say, "should be offered the choice." It is common for people to be told that they 'must' be induced if they are not in labour within 24 hours of their waters breaking and sometimes even sooner, but this is for the individual to decide.

In most cases of PROM labour starts soon after the waters break. Research studies have found that 60–95% of labours begin spontaneously within

24 hours (Hannah 1997, Enkin 2000, Middleton 2017). Almost 90% of mothers will be in spontaneous labour within 48 hours of PROM (Enkin 2000) and 95–98% within 72 hours (Hannah 1996, Enkin 2000).

Since we know that stress hormones slow the progress of labour (Buckley 2011) it's probably helpful, if your waters have broken at term but your contractions have not started, to put the question of induction out of your mind for the time being, and try to relax and stay as calm as possible. This may help your body move into active labour before you need to decide about induction. *(See "What may help an induction to work?" p.128.)*

If your labour hasn't started after 24 hours you can decide whether you want to wait a bit longer or accept induction. If you decide to wait, the NICE guidelines suggest you check for signs of infection by taking your temperature every four hours and checking for an unpleasant-smelling discharge from your vagina. Your hospital may suggest having your baby's movements and heartbeat checked at intervals. It's up to you whether you want this, but if you do you can ask for a community midwife to visit you at home to carry out these checks, rather than having the disruption of going to hospital.

Whilst any illness is a concern, it is extremely rare for a baby to die or suffer serious long-term problems as a result of developing an infection after PROM. In one very large trial (Hannah 1996) one baby out of over 5000 in the study died as a result of an infection. The main concern is about infections with Group B Streptococcus (GBS). For a full discussion of the issues around GBS infection in babies see the AIMS publication "Group B Strep Explained."

Infection in the womb (clinical chorioamnionitis) is thought to affect up to 4% of all term pregnancies. Unlike in the past, it is fortunately now very rare for mothers to die from infection after childbirth – less than one in 100,000 in the UK over the period 2014–16, and that is for all types of infection including flu and pneumonia (MBRRACE 2018).

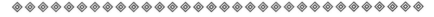

Research Evidence

The NICE Intrapartum care guidelines (NICE 2014, updated 2017) state that the risk of a baby having a serious infection after PROM is 1% compared to 0.5% if the membranes are intact until after labour has started. In other words, normally one in every 200 babies would get an infection during labour but 199 would not; after PROM for every 200 babies, two will have an infection, but 198 will not. However, they do not give a reference for these figures, so it is not clear how good the evidence to back them is. Nor do they say what effect (if any) induction has on the risk.

Further evidence on what effects the risks for you and your baby is discussed below.

What affects the risk of infection in the womb after PROM?
In one large study (Seaward 1997) 4–5% of mothers who had PROM showed some signs of infection if labour began within 24 hours, and 10% if it took between 24 and 48 hours, but there was no further increase if it was more than 48 hours before active labour started.

Risk factor	% of mothers diagnosed
Whole sample	6.7%
No. of vaginal examinations before birth:	
Less than 3	2%
3–4	4%
5–6	7%
7–8	13%
8+	20%
Hours between PROM and labour:	
Under 12	4%
12–24	5%
24–48	10%
Over 48	10%
GBS status:	
Negative or unknown	6.5%
Positive	11%

A greater risk factor was having numerous vaginal examinations between PROM and birth, with over eight examinations raising the risk to 20% (1 in 5). This shows the importance of keeping vaginal examinations to a minimum after PROM – especially as infection in the womb is the biggest risk factor for infection in babies (see below).

The process of induction tends to involve multiple insertions of prostaglandin and multiple internal examinations to check the dilation of the cervix, all of which could make an infection more likely compared with simply waiting at home for labour to start.

Having had a positive test for Group B Streptococcus (GBS) also increased the risk of an infection in the womb, but the authors do not say whether these mothers had antibiotics in labour. *(See "Should you have antibiotics after PROM or Pre-PROM?" p.38.)*

What affects the risk of infection for babies after PROM?

The biggest risk factor for babies appears to be whether there were signs of an infection in the womb (clinical chorioamnionitis) such as a raised temperature during labour, a raised number of white blood cells, or a foul-smelling discharge from the vagina (Seaward 1998). 16% (one in six) of these babies had a "definite or probable infection" but this will have included some (perhaps many) babies who were suspected of having an infection when they didn't.

Risk factor	% of babies with "definite or probable infection"
Whole sample	2.6%
Mother diagnosed with chorioamnionitis	16%
GBS status:	
Negative or unknown	2.3%
Positive	7%
Hours between PROM and labour:	
12–24	2%
24–48	4%
Over 48	4%

The next biggest factor was whether the mother had tested positive for GBS. 7% (about one in 14) of babies born to mothers with GBS-positive status had a "definite or probable infection" but again this does not mean that 7% of their babies had a GBS infection. In the UK early onset GBS infection (which happens in the first week of life) affects one baby in every 1,750 (RCOG 2017).

The study showed no difference in the infection rate whether the delay between PROM and the start of labour was between 24 and 48 hours, or over 48 hours.

Does induction reduce the risk of infection?

The NICE guidelines (NICE 2014, updated 2017) conclusion that induction is appropriate after 24 hours seems to have been made on the basis of the analysis (Seaward 1997, 1998) which showed no increase in infection for mothers or babies if labour starts within 24 hours of PROM, coupled with the evidence that a majority will be in spontaneous labour within 24 hours (Hannah 1997, Enkin 2000, Middleton 2017). However, since rates of infection do not seem to increase any more after 48 hours compared with 24 hours (Seaward 1997, 1998), it's questionable whether there is any great urgency in inducing after 24 hours. It's likely that almost all labours will have begun spontaneously within 48 hours of PROM anyway (Enkin 2000).

The real question is whether induction after PROM is helpful. The available evidence suggests that induction after PROM reduces the time until birth only by about 8–12 hours compared with expectant management (Middleton, 2017). Does that make a difference to the risks? Unfortunately, the evidence that might help us answer this question is limited.

The NICE recommendation was based on a Cochrane review which has since been updated. This newer review (Middleton 2017) combines the results of a number of **randomised controlled trials** but most of these studies had some serious design flaws.

The review authors decided that though induction appeared to reduce the chances of babies being *suspected* of having an infection ("definite or probable infection") there was no clear difference in the chance of them *definitely* having an infection. In fact there may be no real difference in the number of babies infected. The largest trial included (Hannah 1996) found *no* **statistically significant** difference in rates of infection for babies in the expectant management group and those in the induction group.

None of the studies were large enough to show whether there was a statistically significant difference in the number of babies who died around the time of birth, because it was so rare for this to happen – 1–2 in every 1000 babies.

For mothers there was only a small amount of low quality evidence that induction reduces the chances of developing an infection in the womb, from about 11 in every 100 mothers who experienced PROM to about five in every 100. There was no clear difference in the number who had a fever after giving birth.

» » »» » »» » »» » »» » »» » »» » »» » »» » »» » » » »» » » »

Summary

- » It seems that there is probably no increase in the risk of infection for mothers or babies if labour starts spontaneously within 24 hours of PROM, and most labours will.

- » If labour has not started within 24 hours there is some evidence that the risk for both is increased though the **absolute risk** remains small and the majority will not have an infection.

- » It is important to avoid having a lot of internal examinations after PROM, as this increases the risk of infection in the womb more than the time taken for labour to start. As infection in the womb is also the biggest risk factor for the baby, it makes sense to try to keep vaginal examinations to a minimum (or avoid them altogether).

- » There is little if any evidence that induction after PROM is of benefit to babies, and in one large trial (Hannah 1996) it made no difference to the chances of infection.

- » There is some low quality evidence that induction may help to prevent an infection occurring in the womb after PROM. It would be necessary to carry out around 20 inductions to avoid one such infection.

- » The risks of infection after PROM are higher for both baby and mother if the mother has had a positive test for Group B Streptococcus (GBS), but we lack information on the absolute risk in this situation.

~~~~ ~~ ~~~~ ~~ ~~~~ ~~ ~~~~ ~~ ~~~~ ~~ ~~~~

Things to consider

- Do you have a reason for wanting your labour to be induced immediately if you experience PROM (such as knowing you have tested positive for GBS) or are you happy to wait for at least 24 hours for your labour to start?
- If your labour hasn't start within 24 hours of PROM would you prefer to have your labour induced or to wait a bit longer to see if it starts in the next day or so?
- If you decide to wait, for how long would you wait before considering induction (assuming you had no signs of infection)?
- How do you feel about the possible risks of a medical induction and the possibility of needing an unplanned **caesarean** if it fails?
- In what circumstances would you agree to a vaginal examination after PROM, or would you prefer to avoid these altogether?

Preterm Prelabour Rupture of the Membranes (Pre-PROM)

Preterm Prelabour Rupture of the Membranes is defined as the waters breaking before 37 weeks of pregnancy. The issues are similar to PROM, but with the added complication that being born too early carries risks for a baby. It's therefore a matter of trading off the risks of prematurity against the possible increased risk of infection for you and your baby.

The NICE recommendation (NICE 2008) for Pre-PROM says:

- If a woman has preterm prelabour rupture of membranes, induction of labour should not be carried out before 34 weeks unless there are additional obstetric indications (for example, infection or **fetal compromise**).
- If a woman has preterm prelabour rupture of membranes after 34 weeks, the maternity team should discuss the following factors with her before a decision is made about whether to induce labour, using vaginal PGE2:

> » the risks to the woman (for example, sepsis, possible need for caesarean section)
> » the risks to the baby (for example, sepsis, problems relating to preterm birth)
> » the local availability of neonatal intensive care facilities.

Some hospitals may still be working to these guidelines, however RCOG has published a more recent guideline (RCOG 2019) reflecting new research (Bond 2017, discussed below). This new RCOG guideline says, "Women whose pregnancy is complicated by PPROM after 24+0 weeks' gestation and who have no contraindications to continuing the pregnancy should be offered expectant management until 37+0 weeks; timing of birth should be discussed with each woman on an individual basis with careful consideration of patient preference and ongoing clinical assessment." This means that it is better to wait for labour to start rather than having induction after Pre-PROM if there are no other concerns.

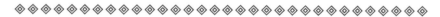

Research Evidence

The NICE **GDG** found very little evidence on which to base their recommendations: three very small trials which seemed to show an increase in infections in the mothers with expectant management, but were not big enough to show if there was a difference in outcomes for the babies, and one observational study which indicated a shorter stay in hospital and less jaundice for babies induced after 34 weeks. The recommendation was therefore not to induce before this apparent "natural break point."

A more recent review (Bond 2017) found no difference between the planned **early birth** and expectant management groups in the number of babies who suffered an infection. However, babies who had a **planned early birth** were more likely to have breathing problems, to need to be ventilated and to need to spend time in a neonatal intensive care unit. They were also more likely to be born by caesarean. The authors concluded that "In women whose waters break before 37 weeks of pregnancy, waiting for labour to begin naturally is the best option for healthier outcomes, as long as there are no other reasons why the baby should be born immediately."

In fact, it seems that most of the expectant management group went into labour within a few days of their waters breaking, as the difference in length of pregnancy between them and the early birth group was only about three days on average.

Having antibiotics during this time was effective in reducing maternal infections. *(See "Should you have antibiotics after PROM or Pre-PROM?", p.38, for a discussion of the pros and cons of antibiotics.)*

There is only one small study that has looked at mothers with Pre-PROM who had tested positive for GBS (Tajik 2014). This wasn't the main purpose of the trial, but the researchers made a chance finding that the risk of babies of GBS-positive mothers developing an infection after Pre-PROM seemed to be lower if the labour was induced immediately, but for GBS-negative mothers there seemed to be no difference. Without more evidence we can't be certain, but this suggests a possible benefit for induction as soon as possible after Pre-PROM if you have tested positive for GBS, however that must be weighed against the higher chance of your baby having breathing problems.

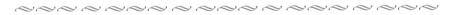

Summary

» The latest evidence supports waiting for labour to begin rather than immediate induction after Pre-PROM, as long as there is no other cause for concern.

» The risk of infection for your baby if you have tested positive for GBS may be reduced if you have immediate induction. However the evidence for this is not strong, and it needs to be balanced against the risks of **premature** birth.

» If you tested negative or have not been tested for GBS there is no evidence that immediate induction is of benefit.

Things to consider

• Have you had a positive test for GBS, or do you have other reasons to suspect that it is present (such as having had a bladder or urine infection during pregnancy)?

• If your hospital recommends immediate induction after Pre-PROM, would you prefer this or to wait for your labour to start?

- If you decide to wait, for how long would you wait before considering induction (assuming you have no signs of infection)?
- How do you feel about the possible risks of a medical induction and the possibility of needing an unplanned **caesarean** if it fails?

Should you have antibiotics after PROM or Pre-PROM?

You may be offered antibiotics to reduce the risk of you or your baby developing an infection after PROM or Pre-PROM.

For babies, the main risk factors for developing an infection after PROM are whether an infection develops in the womb (which would in turn depend on the risk factors discussed above, *see "What affects the risk of infection in the womb after PROM?" p.31*). If you tested positive for GBS during pregnancy or if you develop signs of infection during labour (e.g. raised temperature or offensive-smelling vaginal discharge) you will usually be offered antibiotics.

As with any medical procedure, it is up to you to decide whether you want to take antibiotics.

If you decide to have antibiotics it's usual to have a dose every four hours during labour, given through a cannula (a short, thin tube) which is inserted in your hand or arm. This should make no difference to your ability to move around and use different positions for labour and birth. You should also be able to use a birth pool if you wish, if the end of the tube is taped over and you keep it above the surface of the water. Before you decide whether to take antibiotics you might want to check that you will be supported with your birth choices.

What are the benefits and risks of having antibiotics in labour?

Antibiotics carry some risks. They can have side effects, and a small number of people (including babies) will have an allergic reaction to the drug, so if you have them you should be monitored for this after the first dose is given.

There are also concerns that babies exposed to antibiotics will be less likely to develop a healthy microbiome (the helpful bacteria which normally colonise our bodies), and so more likely to be colonised by harmful bacteria which are antibiotic resistant (Dunn 2017). This could mean that your baby is more likely to develop a gut infection, which can be serious in a newborn. We do not have good research on the long term effects on babies of antibiotics given during labour or at birth.

An interval of more than 24 hours from PROM to the start of labour contractions is one of the risk factors for babies becoming infected with GBS *(see "What affects the risk of infection for babies after PROM?", p.32).* If you have tested positive for GBS or had a GBS infection during this or a previous pregnancy you will probably be offered immediate induction and antibiotics during labour. This is because there is a higher chance of your baby developing a GBS infection compared to the whole pregnant population, just because most of the population will not have GBS in their vaginas and so have very little chance of an infection.

If you have tested negative or not had a test for GBS, and have no signs of infection, there is no convincing evidence that having antibiotics after PROM or Pre-PROM would make any difference to the risk of infection for you or your baby (Wojcieszek 2014, Tajik 2014).

Even if you have tested positive, there is only a small risk that your baby will develop a GBS infection. The Royal College of Obstetricians & Gynaecologists (RCOG 2017) states that having antibiotics during labour reduces the risk of infection from one in 400 to one in 4000, which means that out of every 4000 women with GBS who have antibiotics one baby would still develop an infection but 3999 would not, and for every 4000 mothers who decline antibiotics, ten babies would develop an infection and 3990 would not.

Although GBS infection in babies can be serious, and sadly a small number die of it, most infections that occur are treated successfully. The RCOG leaflet states that of the 43 babies per month (on average) who develop GBS infection in the UK, 38 make a full recovery, three will have long-term disabilities and two die. It is **premature** babies who are at greatest risk; babies born after 37 weeks are much more likely to survive a GBS infection. Not all these cases are associated with PROM, as babies can develop GBS in many other situations as well.

It's estimated that 20–40% of all women have GBS in their vagina at any one time, but most will not know whether they have it there or not as it usually causes no symptoms. It is sometimes found to be present if you have a bladder or urinary tract infection during pregnancy. In the UK routine testing is not recommended. This is because the UK National Screening Committee concluded that the test cannot tell babies who are at risk of GBS infection from those who are not. Routine screening would therefore mean "many thousands of women receiving antibiotics in labour when there is no benefit for them or their babies and the harms this may cause are unknown." However, some people choose to have a test done privately.

Hospitals tend to err on the side of caution and offer antibiotics if GBS was detected at any time in pregnancy, but in fact GBS tends to come and go. The most accurate time for a test to predict whether it will be present at birth is between 35 and 37 weeks of pregnancy. If you decide to have a private test this is the best time to do it. A test done six weeks or more before the birth will incorrectly predict the presence of GBS at birth in 19% of those tested, compared with only 4% if the test is done later. It will also miss as many as 50% of people who are GBS positive at birth, compared to only 13% of mothers tested later (Yancey 1996).

» » »» » »» » »» » »» » »» » »» » »» » »» » »» » »» » »» » » » »» » » »

Summary

» There are some risks in taking antibiotics, including allergic reactions and an increased risk of gut infection in your baby.

» GBS infections are less common and usually less severe in babies born at term than those born prematurely.

» Most GBS infections that occur are identified and treated successfully, but in rare situations they can have serious consequences.

» If you want to be tested for GBS the best time to do this is between 35 and 37 weeks of pregnancy. You will need to arrange this privately.

» **If you have not had a positive test for GBS** and are showing no signs of infection there is no evidence of benefit in you having antibiotics after PROM. You may prefer to decline them, or only have them if you have signs of infection.

» **If you have tested positive for GBS** or have other reasons to think it may be is present (such as a recent infection) there may be a benefit for you and your baby in having antibiotics after PROM. The benefit is greater after Pre-PROM, as premature babies are more likely to be seriously affected by a GBS infection.

» If you prefer to decline antibiotics, the absolute risk of your baby developing an infection is still low.

Things to consider

- Have you had a positive test for GBS, or do you have other reasons to suspect that it is present (such as having had a bladder or urine infection during pregnancy)?

- Do you have any signs that you might be developing an infection in your womb (e.g. a raised temperature or a bad-smelling discharge from your vagina)?

- How do you feel about the risks and benefits for you and your baby of having antibiotics during labour?

What if there is meconium in the waters?

Meconium is the dark, sticky substance which builds up in a baby's bowels during pregnancy. It consists of solid material from the amniotic fluid that your baby has been swallowing. It is usually passed the first time a baby opens their bowels after birth, but in about one in eight labours it is passed during pregnancy or labour (Katz & Bowes 1992).

No one is sure why this happens, but there are three theoretical explanations. One is that the baby's bowels are mature and have become active, which could be particularly likely in a longer pregnancy, and this would not be a cause for any concern. Another is that it could be a sign that the baby has opened her/his bowels in reaction to a short-term stress at some previous time but is not stressed now. Thirdly, it could show that the baby is currently under stress. However, many babies that have heart rate changes indicating stress do not pass meconium, and many that have passed meconium show no other signs of stress. (Unsworth & Vause 2010). In other words, meconium in the waters *might* be, but isn't necessarily, a sign of a baby in distress.

As it's hard to be certain what the cause is, if meconium is found in your waters when they break, you may be encouraged to have an immediate induction, or if your labour has already started to have it **augmented** with an **oxytocin** drip.

If the meconium is thin and brownish in colour it's likely to be 'old' meconium that was passed either because of gut maturity or some stress earlier in pregnancy. If your baby's heartbeat is normal, finding this type of meconium is not an indication of current problems. Thick and greenish or lumpy meconium will probably have been freshly passed. Even so, it is not in itself a sign that your baby is still under stress, and if the heart rate pattern is normal it's unlikely there is a problem.

If there are worrying changes in the heart rate *and* thick meconium is present that makes it more likely that the baby is getting short of oxygen and needs to be born soon (Unsworth & Vause 2010, Davies 2011). The question then is whether induction or **augmentation** is likely to prevent a baby who already appears to be struggling from suffering harm, or whether the sudden strong contractions that induction or augmentation can cause would make it more likely that the baby will become severely distressed. Unfortunately, there is a lack of evidence about this.

Sometimes what are called 'conservative measures' are enough to correct a worrying heart rate. These could include making sure that you are not dehydrated, being reassured and helped to relax, and getting into an upright position. If these are not effective, and your baby seems to be having serious problems then a **caesarean** may be better for them.

The other issue is a rare but serious condition called Meconium Aspiration Syndrome (MAS) which affects about two in 1000 babies and is associated with breathing problems. It's thought that a baby that has become very seriously distressed during labour will sometimes, as a reflex, attempt to gasp, and if this happens when meconium is present, then that will be drawn into the lungs. MAS may therefore be a risk if there is meconium present *and* a baby is suffering severe distress during labour, but it would be unusual for a baby to reach the point where they gasp whilst still in the womb without any warning signs being spotted by a midwife.

It's estimated that 95% of cases of MAS are associated with thick meconium which means it is very rare to see MAS if the meconium is thin.

It is increasingly being questioned whether the presence of meconium in the lungs is what *causes* the breathing problems seen in MAS or whether it is a *result* of them. It may be that low oxygen during labour causes lung damage which then means that the baby is unable to clear meconium from its airways and lungs as it would normally do, rather than the meconium causing the damage (Katz & Bowes 1992).

There is some evidence that the presence of meconium increases the risk of infection after PROM for mothers (Seaward 1997) but it was not found to predict the risk of infection in babies.

For more on this topic, see *www.aims.org.uk/journal/item/troubled-waters.*

» » »» » »» » »» » »» » »» » »» » »» » »» » »» » »» » » » »» » » »

Summary

- » There is no evidence to show whether babies are helped by immediate induction if meconium is found in the waters after PROM, or by augmentation if it's found once labour has begun.
- » If the meconium is thin or looks old and there are no problems with your baby's heartbeat, it's unlikely that your baby is under stress and very unlikely that they will develop MAS, so there seems to be no strong argument for inducing or augmenting the labour.
- » There may be more justification for wanting your baby to be born quickly if there is fresh thick meconium, especially if it is accompanied by heart rate changes that suggest the baby is suffering low oxygen levels.
- » It may be helpful to find ways to relax, move into an upright position and take care of anything that could be contributing to the stress on your baby (such as you being dehydrated) whilst your midwife keeps a careful eye on how your baby is coping.
- » You also have the option of a **caesarean** if you think your baby needs to be born quickly, rather than having an induction or **augmentation**.

Things to consider

- Is this thin or old-looking meconium, or does it look fresh and thick?
- If there is no reason for concern over your baby's well-being other

than the presence of meconium would you want to do something to speed up the birth or prefer to wait and see how things develop?

- How do you feel about the possible risks of induction/augmentation and the possibility of needing an unplanned caesarean if it fails?
- If there is an agreed cause for concern over your baby's well-being and you want her/him to be born quickly, would you prefer to try induction/augmentation or to have a caesarean?

Your age

The AIMS helpline receives many enquiries from pregnant women and people who have been told that they 'must' be induced by 40 weeks, or even earlier, because they are 'older' and there is an increased risk of stillbirth solely because of their age. The age at which someone is defined as 'older' seems to vary between hospitals. In some it is 40 years, in others it is as low as 35 years.

The NICE recommendations on induction to prevent prolonged pregnancy make no distinction between older and younger mothers (NICE 2008).

Stillbirth rates do appear to be higher in those over 40, although it is not known why this is. It does not appear to be due either to their babies being more likely to grow poorly or to a decline in the function of the placenta (RCOG 2013). There isn't currently any way to identify which babies are at risk, and the **absolute risk** is low.

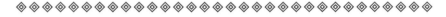

Research Evidence

In the UK the MBRRACE review provides figures for the number of **stillbirths** and **neonatal deaths**. The latest report (MBRRACE 2018) shows that both are higher in mothers over 40 years old compared with younger age groups, but the absolute risk remains low. **Perinatal** deaths occurred in about nine per 1000 mothers aged over 40 compared with an average of just under six per 1000 for those aged between 30 and 39. This means that about 991 mothers out of every 1000 aged over 40 had a baby that survived, compared to 994 out of 1000 of the younger group.

Perinatal deaths per 1000 births

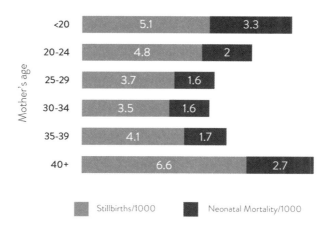

Source: MBRRACE Perinatal Mortality Survey for 12 months to Dec 16

You will see from the graph above that the perinatal death rate for babies of mothers aged 35–39 years was very slightly higher than for those between 20 and 34, but at just under six in 1000 it was actually lower than the rate for those aged 20–24 years (just under seven per 1000). This data therefore does not support the argument for early induction for mothers under 40.

This report groups mothers into convenient five-year sets in order to compare them but what is presumably going on is a gradual increase with age. It is illogical to assume that the risk of perinatal death suddenly jumps up on your 40th birthday.

All of these are figures for the total population and take no account of the fact that the risk for an individual is likely to be affected by things like health, lifestyle factors and socio-economic status. Not all people aged over 40 are the same!

A large population study which analysed over five million health records for mothers in the USA (Reddy 2006) looked at stillbirth rates for women who had already given birth compared with first-time mothers of a similar age. Although there are problems with this type of study (see the AIMS Birth Information web page "Understanding Quantitative Research Evidence", *www.aims.org.uk/information/item/quantitative-research*) it appeared to show that the rates for mothers aged over 35 who had birthed before were lower than for first-time mothers of the same age and in fact lower than for first-time mothers under 35. If this is really the case then there would be no logic in offering early induction to older mothers who have already given birth.

Stillbirths per 1000 births

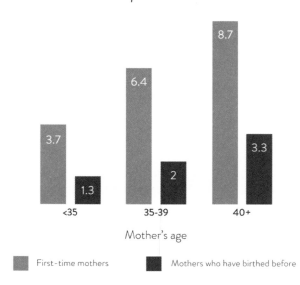

Source: Reddy et al 2006

How does the risk increase with the length of pregnancy?

To answer this question we only have evidence from the above **population study** (Reddy 2006), which also looked at the stillbirth rates at different points in pregnancy for all **ongoing pregnancies**. It reported separately the risk for all mothers and the risk for mothers who did not have any serious medical conditions either before or during pregnancy. The findings for the mothers without medical conditions are shown in the graph below.

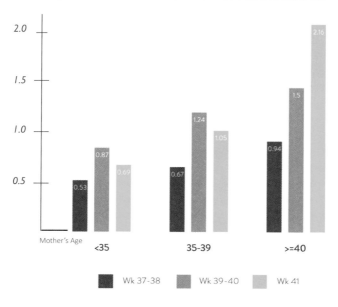

Stillbirths rate per 1000 ongoing pregnancies by length of pregnancy & mother's age (Mothers with no medical conditions)

Source: Reddy et al 2006

For healthy mothers aged 35–39 whose pregnancy lasted between 39 and 40 weeks there was a very small increase in risk (about one additional stillbirth in every 1,750 **ongoing pregnancies**) compared with mothers who birthed at 37 to 38 weeks. There was a slight *decrease* in the proportion who had stillbirths when pregnancy lasted 41 weeks, compared with those who birthed at 39 to 40 weeks.

For healthy mothers aged 40 or over, the stillbirth rate was always higher than it was for younger mothers at the same point in pregnancy, and rose slightly more with the length of pregnancy, but remained low, at 2.2 stillbirths in every 1000 ongoing pregnancies at 41 weeks.

Does induction reduce the risk?

The assumption made by those who recommend induction at 39 or 40 weeks for older pregnant women and people is that it will help to avoid some of the extra stillbirths that can occur in this group. Unfortunately, there is little evidence to tell us whether this is true. It would be difficult to recruit a large enough sample to do a reliable trial for people aged over 35 who have not gone into labour by 40 weeks, as this age group is only about 20% of the birthing population. It would be even harder for those aged over 40, who are about 4% of the total.

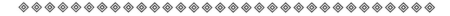

Research Evidence

The little evidence we do have about the effect of induction is from a recent **population study** (Knight, 2017). This used historic UK data to compare the **perinatal death** rate for healthy first-time mothers aged 35 or over who had induction of labour at 39, 40, and 41 weeks of pregnancy, compared with those who had expectant management.

At 39 weeks there was no significant difference in stillbirths or perinatal deaths with induction compared to expectant management, but an increase in the caesarean rate from 29% to 35%.

At 40 weeks induction appeared to reduce perinatal deaths amongst first-time mothers over 35 from 2.6 per 1000 births to 0.8 per 1000. This means that out of 1000 first-time mothers who had an induction at 40 weeks there were approximately two who avoided a perinatal death by doing so, although one in 1000 babies still died. Induction at 40 weeks appeared to increase the chances of a caesarean from 33% to 39% of births.

Unfortunately, this study grouped all women over 35 together, so we can't tell whether the apparent benefit of induction at 40 weeks apples to all of them, or only to a more limited age group. It also tells us nothing about whether there is a benefit for those who have birthed before.

Your doctor may talk about the "35/39 trial" trial of "labor induction in women 35 years of age or older". This trial (Walker 2016) looked at the impact of induction at 39 weeks of pregnancy on *the type of birth* for mothers aged 35 and over, and whether it would increase the caesarean rate. It was never intended to try to detect an effect on stillbirths and doesn't tell us anything about this. (For an interesting review of this trial see Roberts 2019.)

» » »» » »»» » »»» » »»» » »»» » »»» » »»» » »»» » »»» » »»» » » » »»» » » »

Summary

» The one UK **population study** we have (Knight 2017) suggests that there is no benefit to older mothers in having an induction at 39 weeks, but possibly a reduction in **perinatal** deaths (of about 1.8 per 1000 mothers) in having one at 40 weeks.

» The study did not distinguish between those aged 35–39 and those over 40, which means we do not know whether there was the same benefit for the younger age group as the older one. It does not tell us whether there is a benefit for those who have birthed before.

» It also showed that induction at 40 weeks increased the chance of having a **caesarean** from 33% to 39%.

If you are aged 35–39

• The rates of stillbirth and **neonatal death** in the UK are not substantially greater for this age group than those for younger people and in fact are lower than for those aged 20-24.

• The risk of stillbirth for this age group may increase a little more in late pregnancy than it does in younger age groups but there seems to be no increase in the risk between 39/40 weeks and 41 weeks.

- There therefore seems to be no logic for inducing labour at 39 or 40 weeks if you are under 40.
- We have don't have enough evidence to be sure whether early induction would help to reduce stillbirths in this age group.

If you are aged over 40

- In the UK there is a slightly higher risk of a stillbirth or **neonatal death** for this age group than for younger people, though the absolute risk is still low. *(See the graph of MBRRACE data, p.45.)*
- The rate of stillbirth does appear to rise in late pregnancy, possibly 2.2 stillbirths per 1000 **ongoing pregnancies** at 41 weeks compared with about 1.5/1000 at 39/40 weeks, if there are no pre-existing health problems.
- No one knows what causes the higher rate, so there is no way to tell whether a particular baby is at risk purely because of her/his mother's age.
- We don't have enough evidence to be sure whether early induction would help to reduce stillbirths in this age group.

Things to consider

- How might your individual circumstances affect the risks of stillbirth for you, and how do you feel about that level of risk? This may depend on whether you are under or over 40, and whether you have given birth before.
- How do you feel about the possible higher chance of needing an unplanned **caesarean** if you had your labour induced at 39/40 weeks?
- How do you feel about the other possible implications of a medical induction?

- Do you have reason to question the accuracy of the estimated due date in your notes? *(See "How long a pregnancy is 'too long?", p.22 and the AIMS Birth Information web page,* "How accurate is my due date?", *www.aims.org.uk/information/item/due-date.)*

Induction for predicted high birthweight

Babies with a higher than average birthweight are sometimes referred to as **macrosomic** (which means big bodied) or Large for Gestational Age (**LGA**). The definition varies but most hospitals use a birthweight over 4000g (4kg or 8lb 13oz) to define LGA.

If a baby's birthweight is predicted to be this high, it is increasingly common for an induction of labour to be recommended. This is quite a recent trend and the 2008 NICE guidelines on induction state, "In the absence of any other indications, induction of labour should not be carried out simply because a healthcare professional suspects a baby is large for gestational age."

A review of the evidence (Boulvain 2016) published since the NICE guidelines were written may be encouraging doctors to recommend induction, although the evidence of benefit in an otherwise uncomplicated pregnancy is not that strong and of course it is for each person to decide how they feel about the option of induction.

Why is high birthweight a concern?

The main concern regarding high birthweight is that a larger baby may be more likely to experience shoulder dystocia, which is the situation when the baby's head has been born but the shoulders do not follow quickly. There is no clear agreement on when a delay should be classed as shoulder dystocia, but it is estimated to affect six or seven out of every 1000 births (RCOG 2012b). It is an emergency, and naturally very alarming for the parents, but all midwives are trained in a series of manipulations to manage this situation, and in most cases the baby is born within a few minutes and without suffering any lasting harm.

If shoulder dystocia occurs, the first step which your midwife will suggest is to get into a position which will widen the outlet from your pelvis and make it easier for the shoulders to be born. This first step alone works for about 90% of cases (RCOG 2012b) without any further action being needed. Logically, this suggests that shoulder dystocia is less likely to happen, regardless of the size of your baby, if you birth in an upright position, which allows your pelvis to open to its fullest extent. There have been cases of mothers who experienced shoulder dystocia when lying down to give birth but in a later pregnancy birthed a larger baby vaginally when using an upright position.

The most common problem with shoulder dystocia is damage to the nerves in the baby's shoulder (called brachial plexus injury). This affects somewhere between 2% and 16% of all cases of shoulder dystocia though less than 10% of these injuries result in permanent damage (RCOG 2012b). This means that somewhere between two and 16 in every 1000 babies who experience shoulder dystocia will have long-term nerve damage, with the other 998–984 recovering fully.

The other main risk is that the baby will suffer a broken collarbone. A recent review found that 2% of suspected big babies experienced this, but fortunately these injuries usually heal well without long-term consequences (Boulvain 2016).

If the midwife is unable to help the baby to be born quickly enough, the baby may suffer from lack of oxygen which could cause brain damage (e.g. **cerebral palsy**) or even death, but this is very rare. There don't seem to be any published figures for how common these serious outcomes are, probably because they are fortunately too rare to show up in the studies which have been done.

NB: Doctors are probably becoming more careful about informing people about the risks from shoulder dystocia after a court case (Montgomery 2015). In this a doctor was held to be negligent for not discussing the risks with a mother with diabetes whose baby was born with cerebral palsy. It is right that you should be informed of the risks, but some doctors may be focusing on the small risk of a baby suffering brain damage or dying as a result of shoulder dystocia and failing to balance this against the risks of interventions. (For more about the Montgomery case see *www.aims.org.uk/journal/item/montgomery*.)

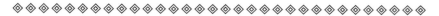

Research Evidence

The main evidence is from a **meta-analysis** (Boulvain 2018) which included four randomised controlled trials but was dominated by one trial where labour was induced between 37 and 38+6 weeks.

It found some evidence described as 'moderate quality' that early induction for suspected big babies reduced the rate of shoulder dystocia, and some higher quality evidence that it reduced the number of babies with broken collarbones, but the studies were too small to show a difference in such rare events as a nerve injury or of a baby not getting enough oxygen during the birth.

The absolute risk of shoulder dystocia was 41 out of 1000 babies when labour was induced compared to 68 out of 1000 with expectant management. In other words, induction does not remove the risk of shoulder dystocia but may help about 27 out of every 1000 **LGA** babies to avoid it. When the mothers chose to wait 932 babies out of 1000 were born without shoulder dystocia, compared with 959 when labour was induced.

In the induction group four babies out of 1000 suffered a fracture, compared to twenty out of 1000 in the group who waited.

Induction increased the number of mothers who had severe tears in their perineum (the area at the back of the vagina) from seven in 1000 without induction to 27 in 1000. The number of babies who needed to have treatment for jaundice increased from 70 in 1000 to 110 in 1000 with induction.

The review concludes that "Although some parents and doctors may feel the existing evidence is sufficient to justify inducing labour, others may disagree." In other words, the evidence is not conclusive, and parents need to decide for themselves and have that decision supported.

Can shoulder dystocia be predicted?

Carrying a baby with an estimated birthweight of over 4000g (8lb 13 oz) seems to increase the likelihood of shoulder dystocia, however the estimated size of the baby is not a very good way of predicting whether this complication will occur.

There are other factors which are thought to be associated with a higher chance of shoulder dystocia, but statistical modelling has shown that these are also not good at predicting whether it will happen (RCOG 2012b):

- having diabetes,
- having a body mass index (BMI) of over 30 kg/m2, or
- having had a previous experience of shoulder dystocia.

People with any of these risk factors are often told they have a 'choice' between early induction and a planned caesarean, but they also have the right to wait for spontaneous labour if they choose. *(See "What is the risk of shoulder dystocia?", p.60.)*

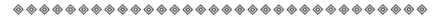

Research Evidence

RCOG says "There is a relationship between fetal size and shoulder dystocia, but it is not a good predictor: partly because fetal size is difficult to determine accurately, but also because the large majority of infants with a birth weight of ≥4500g do not develop shoulder dystocia. Equally important, 48% of births complicated by shoulder dystocia occur with infants who weigh less than 4000g." (RCOG 2012b). In other words, not only is it very hard to tell with any accuracy how big a baby is going to be at birth, but most large babies – even if over 4500g (9lb 15oz) – are born without any difficulty. Also, almost half of all cases of shoulder dystocia occur in babies that weigh less than 4000g.

Shoulder dystocia seems to have become more common in recent decades. This may be due in part to an increase in the number of **LGA** (Large for Gestational Age) babies, though a recent review (Menticoglou 2018) suggests it could also be due to "the increased use of **epidural** anaesthesia … It is certainly plausible that a woman unencumbered by epidural anaesthesia and allowed to assume her own position for pushing would probably be able to push the shoulders out more easily."

Induction itself is listed as a risk factor for shoulder dystocia so could potentially cause the problem it was intended to prevent. This might be because when labour is induced it is common to have continuous monitoring and an **epidural**, both of which could affect the position that is used for birth.

A recent review of the evidence (Bingham 2010) found that 12% of mothers who had previously experienced shoulder dystocia had the same problem in subsequent pregnancies. That means that about one in eight such mothers would experience shoulder dystocia again. However, this may not be true for all mothers as the review does not tell us how many of the women also had diabetes, a high BMI or a tendency to grow large babies, nor the position the mothers were in for the birth, any of which might have affected their risks in both the first and later pregnancies.

How is high birthweight predicted?

A midwife will offer to measure how your bump is growing through pregnancy, and to plot the measurements on a **fetal growth chart**. If the chart suggests that your baby is going to be larger than average, she will probably recommend an ultrasound scan to check.

Measuring with a tape measure is not always accurate, but if you see the same midwife each time you will probably get a more accurate picture of how your baby is growing than if you see lots of different midwives.

An ultrasound may be suggested if the measurement is over the 90th centile of the chart. This is the estimated weight which 90% of babies are expected to be below, so there will always be one in 10 babies who are over the 90th centile (and one in 20 over the 95th). For some people this will just be part of the normal variation seen in any population – for example, taller parents are likely to have larger babies.

Standard **growth charts** take no account of factors which can affect your baby's size such as your height, weight and ethnic heritage, and so some NHS Trusts have introduced customised charts (GROW charts) which try to adjust for this. It is thought that these should be more accurate than the standard growth charts. The GROW charts are mainly designed to identify babies that are growing poorly, but anecdotally it seems that they may be resulting in more people being told that they have a big baby.

It can also happen that if you are having an ultrasound scan in late pregnancy for some other reason (such as checking whether a low-lying placenta has moved out of the way) you will be told that the scan suggests a big baby and that you ought to consider induction.

Does ultrasound estimate birthweight accurately?

It is widely recognised that the size of a baby in late pregnancy is "difficult to determine accurately" (RCOG 2012b). Ultrasound scans carried out in the third trimester can over- or underestimate the actual birthweight by as much as 10%. This means that a baby who is predicted to have a birthweight of 4000g could weigh between 3600g and 4400g at birth. As the main study on late pregnancy ultrasound estimates states, an ultrasound may be "moderately useful" in identifying big babies and rather less good at ruling out the possibility of a big baby, but "over-reliance on them to guide practice should be avoided" (Coomarasamy 2005). In other words, one scan finding in late pregnancy doesn't necessarily mean that much.

If your midwife has previously found no cause for concern or if the ultrasound predicted weight is only just over the cut-off point for LGA, it's questionable whether a decision about induction should be made based on a single ultrasound estimate. In these situations, you might want to ask for a repeat growth scan in a week or so (depending how far advanced your pregnancy is) to see if the finding is confirmed – though the same possibility of a 10% over- or underestimation in birthweight would still apply.

You may also want to consider your own and your family's history. If you or your relatives have previously birthed larger than average babies without problems you may feel less concerned about birthing (another) baby weighing over 4kg.

» » »» » »» » »» » »» » »» » »» » »» » »» » »» » » » »» » » »

Summary

- » The prediction of whether your baby is likely to have a high birthweight may be more accurate if a customised GROW chart that takes account of your height, weight and ethnic heritage is used.
- » Ultrasound scans in late pregnancy are known to be of limited accuracy. If the recommendation for induction is based on a single scan result, you may want to wait and have a repeat scan to check but the 10% margin of error will still apply.
- » Most vaginal births of babies who are predicted to weigh over 4000g are unaffected by shoulder dystocia.
- » Estimated birthweight is not a good way of predicting whether it will occur. Estimates are not very accurate, and about half of all cases of shoulder dystocia occur with babies who are smaller than 4000g.
- » In most cases of shoulder dystocia, the baby is born quickly and suffers no harm.
- » The main risks if shoulder dystocia occurs are that the baby will have a broken collarbone or that there will be damage to the nerves in their shoulder. Most of these injuries heal well and there is no long-term harm. Much more rarely, if there is a long delay, a baby may suffer brain damage or even die.
- » There is some evidence of moderate quality that induction reduces (though does not remove) the chances of a baby who weighs over 4000g experiencing shoulder dystocia and/or a broken collar-bone. There isn't enough evidence to show whether induction makes a difference to nerve injuries or the more serious outcomes associated with shoulder dystocia, probably because they are too rare to show up in studies.
- » There are some increased risks from induction for a suspected large baby including more chance of a severe tear in the perineum and more babies needing treatment for jaundice.

» The risk of shoulder dystocia is probably higher for people who also have one or more additional risk factors such as diabetes, a high BMI or a previous shoulder dystocia.

(For more about the risks if you have diabetes see "What is the risk of shoulder dystocia?", p.60.)

Things to consider

- Is your baby suspected to be large based on a single ultrasound scan in late pregnancy?
- Has your midwife previously expressed any concerns about the size of your baby?
- If you are uncertain about the accuracy of the birthweight estimate, or if it is borderline, do you want another ultrasound scan to check before you decide about early induction?
- Do you have any risk factors for shoulder dystocia other than a suspected high birthweight (i.e. diabetes, a high BMI or a previous shoulder dystocia)?
- Have you or your relatives previously birthed larger than average babies without problems?
- If the only concern is a suspected high birthweight, how do you feel about the possible risks and benefits of an induction in this situation, or would you prefer to wait for your labour to start if there are no other concerns about you or your baby's well-being?
- If you have other risk factors, how do you feel about the options of induction or **caesarean**, or waiting for your labour to start if there are no other concerns about you or your baby's well-being?

Diabetes and predicted high birthweight

There are two main reasons why induction may be recommended for pregnancies affected by diabetes.

1. A slightly higher chance of stillbirth in late pregnancy.
2. Poorly-controlled blood glucose leading to a Large for Gestational Age (**LGA)** baby and a higher risk of shoulder dystocia.

The evidence suggests that the risks of stillbirth and consequences for recommended timing of birth are different for pregnant women and people who develop diabetes in the course of their pregnancy (gestational diabetes mellitus or GDM for short) and for those who already have type 1 or type 2 diabetes before becoming pregnant, so we are discussing them separately.

The research on the risks of having an LGA baby and of shoulder dystocia does not distinguish between mothers with different forms of diabetes, so we consider them together.

What is the risk of shoulder dystocia if you have diabetes?

For more about shoulder dystocia and the risk factors for it, see *"Induction for predicted high birthweight" p.52.*

According to a recent review (Menticoglou 2018) "Women with diabetes have about a 20% chance of delivering a baby [weighing] more than four kg". This means that 20 out of 100 mothers with diabetes are likely to have an LGA baby compared to 10 out of 100 in the total population (ONS 2017).

The RCOG guidelines (RCOG 2012b) state that babies of diabetic mothers have somewhere between two and four times the chance of experiencing shoulder dystocia compared with a baby of the same birth weight whose mother did not have diabetes. This is based on two **population studies** (Nesbit 1998, Acker 1985) which only looked at mothers with diabetes whose babies weighed over 4000g.

These studies suggest that for a predicted birthweight between 4000 and 4500g the risk of a mother with diabetes experiencing shoulder dystocia is probably between 8% and 12%. If the birthweight is predicted to be over 4500g the risk may be as high as 20% or more. For this reason if you have diabetes and your baby appears LGA you may be advised to have a caesarean rather than an induction, especially if the predicted birthweight is over 4500g. A recent legal case (Montogomery) has said that mothers with diabetes should be informed of these higher risks.

National Service Framework for Diabetes says that "Tight blood glucose control during the third trimester can reduce the risk of fetal **macrosomia** and its associated consequences." This suggests that if you have a well-controlled blood glucose level the chances of having an LGA baby and the associated increased risk of shoulder dystocia should be lower than if it is poorly controlled. A review (Martis 2018) concluded that lifestyle changes including healthy eating, physical activity and self-monitoring of blood sugar level *may* result in fewer LGA babies being born to mothers with **GDM**, though these lifestyle interventions also appeared to increase the number of inductions. However, the evidence for this was not very strong. The review did not consider those with type 1 or type 2 diabetes.

» » »» » »» » »» » »» » »» » »» » »» » »» » »» » »» » » » »» » » »

Summary

  » Your risk of shoulder dystocia if your baby is predicted to be LGA will be higher than for someone with a similar-sized baby who is not diabetic.

  » You may be advised to have a **caesarean**, especially if the predicted birthweight is over 4500g (9lb 14oz).

  » Good blood glucose control in pregnancy may help to reduce the risk of having an LGA baby.

Gestational Diabetes Mellitus (GDM)

For more information on the topic of GDM in pregnancy, including issues around testing and management, you might like to look at the AIMS book, "Gestational Diabetes", www.aims.org.uk/shop/item/gestational-diabetes.

For concerns over having a large baby, see "What is the risk of shoulder dystocia if you have diabetes?", p.60.

The NICE Guideline on Diabetes in pregnancy (NICE 2015b) recommends in order to reduce the risk of stillbirth:

- Advise women with gestational diabetes to give birth no later than 40+6 weeks, and offer elective birth (by induction of labour, or by caesarean section if indicated) to women who have not given birth by this time.
- Consider elective birth before 40+6 weeks for women with gestational diabetes if there are maternal or fetal complications.

There is some limited evidence that the stillbirth rate in pregnancies affected by GDM is somewhat higher than average and may start to rise more steeply after 41 weeks, although the absolute risk remains low.

There is no good evidence that induction or planned caesarean is beneficial for those with GDM if their blood glucose is well controlled either by diet or drugs and they have no other complicating factors.

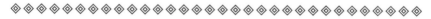

Research Evidence

The NICE recommendation to give birth no later than 40 weeks and six days is based on a single US population study (Rosenstein 2012). There are problems with relying on this type of research (see the AIMS Birth Information web page "Understanding Research Evidence", *www.aims.org.uk/information/item/quantitative-research*) and maternity care in the USA is very different from that in the UK, but at least this study looked at a very large number of women.

It found that the stillbirth risk for mothers with GDM was slightly higher than for other mothers from 36 to 41 weeks (though actually a bit lower at 42 weeks). It rose from just over five in every 10,000 **ongoing pregnancies** at 40 weeks to about eight in 10,000 at 41 weeks. For comparison, the rates in mothers without GDM rose from just under five in 10,000 at 40 weeks to about six in 10,000 at 41 weeks, so the difference between mothers with and without GDM was extremely small.

The rate of **neonatal deaths** for mothers with GDM was consistently a little lower than for those without. The authors did not quote **perinatal** death rates, but it looks as though these may have followed a similar pattern.

Unfortunately, the study does not differentiate between women with GDM whose blood glucose levels were well controlled and those which were not, nor does it take account of other health or lifestyle figures which might differ between these groups, so we don't know whether the earlier rise in stillbirth rate applies to everyone with GDM or only to those with other risk factors.

The NICE **GDG** concluded on the basis of the Rosenstein study that "Given that avoidance of stillbirth was the philosophy underpinning the timing of delivery, the group felt that in women with uncomplicated gestational diabetes, elective delivery could be delayed until 40+6 days." This contrasts with what has been the practice of inducing these mothers by 40 weeks.

Does induction reduce the risk?

There is almost no evidence on the question of whether induction at 40+6 days as NICE recommends for pregnancies affected by GDM is of any benefit in reducing stillbirths. What little there is suggests that very large numbers of inductions would be needed to prevent one stillbirth.

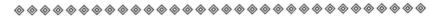

Research Evidence

The authors of the Rosenstein study compared the rate of infant deaths in a given week of pregnancy with the rate of stillbirth in that week plus the rate of infant death in the following week. This was intended to mimic the effect of induction in that week versus expectant management for one further week, but it doesn't prove that induction would make a difference. They estimated that it would be necessary to induce 1300 people at 40 weeks to avoid one death. At 41 weeks the difference was not statistically significant.

The GDG found only three small studies which looked directly at induction versus expectant management in mothers with GDM, and there has since been another one, but they were all far too small to detect whether induction affected the stillbirth rate because stillbirths are so rare (Kjos 1993, Lurie 1996, Alberico 2010, Alberico 2017).

The GDG also commented that "Evidence was much less robust that for women with gestational diabetes adverse pregnancy outcomes, apart from mortality, were related to the timing of birth." In other words, there is even less evidence than for stillbirth that induction has other health benefits for mother or baby.

A review (Biesty 2018a) published since the guideline was issued similarly concluded that "There is insufficient evidence to clearly identify if there are differences in health outcomes for women with gestational diabetes and their babies when elective birth is undertaken compared to waiting for labour to start spontaneously or until 41 weeks' gestation if all is well."

In other words, there seems to be no case for induction or planned caesarean before 41 weeks for otherwise healthy mothers with well-controlled blood glucose levels and whose babies are growing normally. There is no evidence for induction after 41 weeks either.

» » »» » »» » »» » »» » »» » »» » »» » »» » »» » »» » » » »» » » »

Summary

   » There is some limited evidence having GDM may increase the risk of stillbirth from about five in every 10,000 **ongoing pregnancies** at 40 weeks to about eight in 10,000 at 41 weeks but it may fall slightly after that. The absolute risk is low, and the best available estimate is that it would be necessary for about 1300 people with GDM to have induction at 40 weeks in order to avoid one stillbirth.

   » The few studies that have been done comparing induction for GDM with **expectant management** were much too small to detect any difference in stillbirth rates, and most failed to find any reduction in the percentage of LGA babies.

   » There seems to be no good evidence to tell us whether early induction for women with GDM would help to avoid any stillbirths.

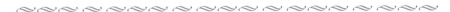

Things to consider

   • Is your blood-glucose level well controlled?
   • Is your baby growing at a normal rate?
   • Are there any reasons for concern about your baby's well-being other than that you have tested positive for GDM?

- How confident are you that the test result was accurate?
- How do you feel about the possible risks of a medical induction and the possibility of needing an unplanned **caesarean** if it fails?

Type 1 or 2 diabetes

The main concerns which might lead to a recommendation of induction for mothers and pregnant people with type 1 or type 2 diabetes are the same as for people who develop it for the first time during pregnancy (GDM), but the recommended timings are different. *(See also "What is the risk of shoulder dystocia?", p.60.)*

Note that we are not considering other health issues for babies in pregnancies affected by type 1 or type 2 diabetes, which are outside the scope of this book.

The NICE guidelines on diabetes in pregnancy (NICE 2015b) recommend:

- Advise pregnant women with type 1 or type 2 diabetes and no other complications to have an elective birth by induction of labour, or by elective caesarean section if indicated, between 37+0 weeks and 38+6 weeks of pregnancy.
- Consider elective birth *before* 37+0 weeks for women with type 1 or type 2 diabetes if there are metabolic or any other maternal or fetal complications.

The GDG say that 37 weeks was *intended as a minimum* for those with uncomplicated type 1 or type 2 diabetes and they "hoped that, in practice, this would result in such women being routinely offered elective delivery nearer 38+6 weeks than 37+0." This was to avoid unnecessary **pre-term** or **early term** births, which increase the risks the baby (such as breathing problems and admission to special care) as well as the risks of a failed induction of labour and a caesarean.

Unfortunately, the evidence about how the stillbirth risk changes with length of pregnancy in people with type 1 or type 2 diabetes is very limited and of poor quality.

In the UK more than half of births to mothers with pre-existing diabetes take place between 37 and 39 weeks, in line with the guidelines. (NPID 2016), but 43% of those with type 1 and 21% with type 2 diabetes birthed before 37 weeks, and there is huge variation in this around the country. Less than one in six went into labour spontaneously and those who had their labours induced had a high chance of having an unplanned caesarean (47% of type 1 and 36% of type 2 if induced before 37 weeks; 34% and 29% respectively if after 38 weeks.)

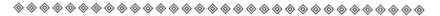

Research Evidence

The NICE guidelines are based on one UK population study (Holman 2014) which analysed the records of mothers with and without pre-existing diabetes. There are problems with relying on this type of study (see the AIMS Birth Information web page "Understanding Quantitative Research Evidence", *www.aims.org.uk/information/ item/quantitative-research)* but this is the only evidence we have.

According to the **GDG**'s analysis of this study the stillbirth rate for women with type 1 or type 2 diabetes was at its lowest at 37–38+6 weeks (about five per 1000 mothers) and this was not significantly different to the rate for all mothers in England and Wales. From 39 weeks it rose to 11 per 1000 mothers, compared with 1.5 per 1000 for all mothers birthing at that point. Based on this finding the GDG recommend that "such women should be offered elective delivery by 38+6 weeks."

There is, however, no evidence to show whether early induction because of pre-existing diabetes reduces the risk of stillbirth because no good quality studies have been done (Biesty 2018b). It would probably be almost impossible to carry out a large enough study to show a significant difference. The population study described above did not report separately on outcomes for mothers who did or did not have their labours induced at a particular stage of pregnancy, so we don't know how that might have affected the observed stillbirth rates.

Summary

» The risk of stillbirth seems to be higher for those with type 1 or type 2 diabetes than for the population as a whole.

» There is limited evidence for how the risk changes through pregnancy. It appears to be similar to the rest of the population at 37–38 weeks but to rise substantially after 39 weeks. This is why the NICE guidelines recommend offering induction or caesarean by 38 weeks and six days.

» We do not know whether induction at this point improves the outcome for babies of mothers with pre-existing diabetes as there is no good evidence on this.

» There is a high chance of having an unplanned caesarean if you have type 1 or type 2 diabetes and have your labour induced.

Things to consider

- Is your blood-glucose level well controlled?
- Is your baby growing at a normal rate?
- Are there any reasons for concern about your baby's well-being other than that you have pre-existing diabetes?
- How do you feel about the increase in stillbirth risk if your pregnancy lasts more than 39 weeks?
- How do you feel about the risks of a medical induction and the possibility of needing an unplanned **caesarean** if it fails?

Baby's well-being

There are various situations where induction may be suggested because of concerns about a baby's well-being. In this chapter we consider three common ones – poor suspected growth, low amniotic fluid (oligohydramnios) and high amniotic fluid (polyhydramnios).

How might this affect the timing of the birth?

If there is a serious concern about your baby's well-being your midwife or doctor may recommend an early birth by induction or caesarean.

As discussed in *"Deciding about induction before 39 weeks" p.13,* early birth carries some risks, especially for **premature** babies. Even **early term** babies (born between 37 and 39 weeks) are more likely to experience health problems including breathing difficulties than those born after 39 weeks (ACOG 2013), so if the problem is not severe and does not worsen, some people will choose to wait at least till 37 or till 39 weeks.

Your decision about whether to bring the birth forward, and whether to have induction or a planned caesarean, may therefore depend on how many weeks pregnant you are, the current health of your baby and how severe the problem seems to be. **It's important to get clear information on these points from your doctors and midwives**.

Questions to ask

Faced with a decision about whether to give birth early because of concerns about your baby you need your midwives and doctors to give you information about your specific situation so that you can weigh up the risks and benefits of the different options. The things you might want to ask include:

- How certain is the diagnosis? (If it is border line it might be worth asking to be retested before making any decision.)
- How serious does the problem seem to be?

- What warning signs might mean that the condition is worsening?
- What are the possible risks to my baby of continuing the pregnancy, at least up to a certain point (e.g. to 37or 39 weeks)? How would my baby's well-being be monitored during this time?
- If my baby was born **prematurely** or at **early term**, what are the possible risks or other consequences of that? What care might be needed once they were born?
- What are the risks, benefits, and likelihood of success, of an induction in this situation, at this stage of pregnancy?
- What are the risks and benefits of a caesarean for me and my baby?

Suspected low amniotic fluid (oligohydramnios)

Induction may be advised if an ultrasound scan in late pregnancy suggests that the volume of the waters around your baby (the amniotic fluid) has fallen too low. Low amniotic fluid is known as oligohydramnios and it is thought to occur in between one and five in 100 pregnancies at term (Leeman 2005).

Sometimes this is a sign of a problem which might itself be a reason for planning an early birth, such as **pre-eclampsia**, the baby growing poorly or a problem with the baby's kidneys. If so, the oligohydramnios is **a symptom and not a cause** of the problems. Often there is no obvious medical cause and then it is more questionable whether an induction is helpful. It appears to be normal for the volume of the amniotic fluid to decrease towards the end of pregnancy, and this may be part of the mechanism for initiating labour (Sherer 2001). It is not at all clear how much of a reduction is 'too much'.

Ultrasound measurement of amniotic fluid volume in late pregnancy is problematic, and neither of the two common methods used is very accurate. For the 'amniotic fluid index' (AFI) the sonographer measures the diameter of the largest pocket of fluid in each quarter of the womb and adds these figures up. For the 'single deepest vertical pocket' method, they look at the measurements of the largest pocket of fluid that they can see. For both methods, different people seem to use different figures as the cut-off for diagnosing oligohydramnios, which adds to the confusion.

A review of these two methods concluded that using AFI results in more diagnoses of oligohydramnios, more inductions and more caesareans but without there being any improvement in the outcomes for babies (Nabhan 2008). In other words, AFI led to more unnecessary interventions. If you are told you have oligohydramnios you might want to check which method has been used to measure it.

It is also worth checking whether the measurement is borderline, and whether it is a one-off finding or short-term variation before making any decision. The measurement can be affected by being dehydrated, by the pressure the operator uses while performing the ultrasound scan and by the position the baby is in (Nabhan 2008). It's also not uncommon for oligohydramnios to be diagnosed when a baby has a full bladder as the volume of fluid in the bladder is therefore not being included in the amniotic fluid measurement. All of this means that a single scan is not very reliable. Oligohydramnios can often be corrected very quickly by drinking more fluid (Leeman 2005).

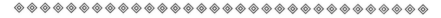

Research Evidence

Historically, oligohydramnios has been associated with an increase in poor health outcomes for babies, but these findings would have included babies with birth defects or poor growth and mothers with underlying medical conditions (Sherer 2001). If any of these problems is present there may be a reason for considering early birth, but there is no evidence that a finding of oligohydramnios is by itself is a reason for induction.

One review of the available evidence (Shrem 2016) found that mothers with mild oligohydramnios and no other obvious problem were significantly more likely to have their labours induced, to have a caesarean and/or for their babies to be admitted to intensive care, but it wasn't any more likely that their babies would show signs of distress during labour.

In the one small **randomised controlled trial** (Ek 2005) which has compared induction with **expectant management** for mothers with oligohydramnios there was no difference in any of the health outcomes for mothers or babies, though it was too small a study to show a difference in rare outcomes such as stillbirth.

» » »» » »» » »» » »» » »» » »» » »» » »» » »» » »» » » » »» » » »

Summary

» It seems likely that the increasing frequency with which mothers are having ultrasound scans in late pregnancy is leading to oligohydramnios being over-diagnosed.

» There may be an underlying cause such as **pre-eclampsia**, the baby growing poorly or a problem with the baby's kidneys.

» In the absence of any obvious cause it may be part of the natural preparation for labour, or a short-term variation which can be corrected very quickly by drinking more fluid (Leeman 2005).

» There is no evidence that a finding of oligohydramnios in the absence of any other concerns about mother or baby's health is a reason for induction.

» Mothers with oligohydramnios are more likely to have their labours induced which may result in more caesareans, but there is no evidence that this benefits them or their babies if there are no other reasons for concern.

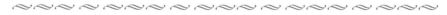

Things to consider

- Which method was used to measure your amniotic fluid volume?
- Was the measurement borderline?
- Could you have been dehydrated at the time?
- Are there any signs of health problems for you or your baby?

- Would you like to have the measurement repeated before you take any decision?
- Would you like other tests of your baby's well-being to be done before you decide?

Also see "Baby's well-being – questions to ask" p.68.

Suspected high amniotic fluid (polyhydramnios)

The opposite of the previous situation is polyhydramnios, where the volume of the waters around your baby (the amniotic fluid) appears to be unusually large. Sometimes this is picked up following a routine antenatal appointment where a midwife suspects a big baby, but an ultrasound scan then suggests that it is extra fluid causing the bump to measure large. Alternatively, it may be diagnosed when an ultrasound scan is done in late pregnancy for some other reason.

There is no evidence-based agreement about what level is 'too high' and no understanding of how the level normally changes as pregnancy progresses (Magann 2011).

As explained in the previous section on low amniotic fluid, the measurement of amniotic fluid levels in late pregnancy is not very accurate, and different hospitals may use different methods and cut-off points for diagnosing polyhydramnios. Probably as a result of these factors, estimates for how common it is range from 0.2% to 3.9% of all pregnancies (Karkhanis 2014).

According to the NHS England website "Most women with polyhydramnios won't have any significant problems during their pregnancy and will have a healthy baby. You can usually wait for labour to start naturally. Sometimes induction (starting labour with medication) or a caesarean section (an operation to deliver your baby) may be needed if there's a risk to you or your baby."

There are no specific guidelines about induction for polyhydramnios alone, so your decision needs to take account of the severity of the condition and whether there is an underlying health problem which is causing it. Sometimes there is an identifiable reason such as uncontrolled diabetes, an infection or a birth defect (especially those that affect the baby's ability to swallow), but for 50–60% of cases of polyhydramnios there is no obvious cause (Karkhanis 2014).

You can ask your midwife or doctor whether your polyhydramnios is classed as mild or severe, and whether there appears to be an underlying cause, so that you can have an informed discussion about what that means for the timing of the birth. If there is no obvious cause, you might want to ask whether there are any further investigations that can be done to try to detect one.

Mild polyhydramnios with no obvious cause is associated with a higher chance of having a large baby but does not seem to be associated with any health problems for the baby (Smith 1992).

Severe unexplained polyhydramnios does seem to be associated with more stillbirths and babies who are born in poor condition.

The other concerns with severe polyhydramnios are that it could cause complications for the birth *(see "Severe polyhydramnios: possible birth complications", p.74)*, and pre-term birth seems to be more common.

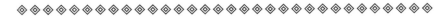

Research Evidence

An underlying cause is found in only about one in five cases of mild polyhydramnios, but in nine out of ten cases of moderate to severe polyhydramnios (Hamza 2013).

There is no evidence about whether induction for polyhydramnios alone, in the absence of other concerns, is of benefit (Karkhanis 2014) and certainly for mild polyhydramnios there seems to be no compelling reason to intervene if all is well otherwise.

If the cause of the polyhydramnios can be identified then that may or may not be a reason for suggesting that the baby is born early, depending on individual circumstances.

Severe polyhydramnios: possible birth complications

'Unstable lie'

If there is a lot of fluid, then a baby may stay floating high in the womb instead of moving down into the pelvis in late pregnancy or early labour. This can lead to what's called an 'unstable lie', where the baby keeps changing position and so may be 'transverse' (lying horizontally across the womb) during labour. A transverse baby cannot be born vaginally so if they cannot be turned during labour would need to be born by **caesarean**.

Cord prolapse

If the waters break when the baby's head is not well engaged (well down in the pelvis), there is a slight risk that the cord will be washed down and through the cervix. This situation (cord prolapse) is uncommon, but when it happens it is an emergency and the baby usually needs to be born quickly by **caesarean**, though occasionally, if the cervix is fully dilated, it is possible to give birth vaginally (RCOG 2015c).

Cord prolapse is unpredictable and can happen to anyone. It is estimated to affect somewhere between one and five in 1000 births overall but may be more common with severe polyhydramnios and/or if the baby is lying breech (bottom first) or transverse, or is head down but has not engaged (RCOG 2015c).

If you have polyhydramnios and your baby is lying transverse or has an unstable lie, you may be recommended to stay in hospital from 37 weeks of pregnancy, so that if a cord prolapse occurs it can be dealt with quickly. Alternatively, or in addition, you may be recommended to have your labour induced and let your midwife or doctor break the waters in a 'controlled' way while trying to hold your baby in a head-down position. This may also be recommended if you have polyhydramnios and are having an induction for some other reason. There is a risk that the induction itself might cause a cord prolapse (RCOG 2015c) and it is up to you whether you want it to be done. You might prefer to wait and see whether your baby moves into a better position by the start of your labour and then decide what to do.

Placental abruption

This is when the placenta starts to detach from the wall of the womb either during pregnancy or labour. It's estimated to affect up to one in 100 pregnancies to some extent and can happen in any pregnancy. It is thought that polyhydramnios may increase the chances of it occurring if, when the waters break, there is a sudden change in pressure inside the womb. There seems to be no hard evidence for how common this is, but it's likely that it's more of a problem if the volume of fluid is very high. For more about placental abruption see *www.babycentre.co.uk/a1024974/placental-abruption*.

» » »»» » »»» » » »»» » »»» » »»» » »»» » »»» » »»» » »»» » » » »»» » » »

Summary

» There is no evidence-based agreement about what level of amniotic fluid is 'too high' and no understanding of how the level normally changes as pregnancy progresses (Magann 2011).

» *Mild polyhydramnios* with no obvious cause is associated with a higher chance of having a large baby but does not seem to be associated with any health problems for the baby (Smith 1992). There is no evidence for recommending induction in this situation if there is no other cause for concern.

» *Severe polyhydramnios* usually has a detectable underlying cause which may be the main factor in deciding about options for the birth.

» *Severe polyhydramnios* probably increases the chances of birth complications such as **premature** labour, transverse or unstable lie, cord prolapse and placental abruption, but it's not clear how much it increases these risks or exactly what level of polyhydramnios should give cause for concern.

» There is no evidence to show whether if there are no other causes for concern induction would improve the outcome, even if the polyhydramnios is severe.

Things to consider

- Is the level of polyhydramnios mild or severe?
- Is there any obvious reason for the high fluid volume?
  - » If so, you might want to ask about the consequences of that underlying condition for the timing of the birth and the health of you and your baby
  - » If not, you might want to ask what further investigations, if any, could be done to try to detect the cause.
- If your baby is lying transverse or has an unstable lie, how would you feel about being in hospital from 37 weeks?
- If you have severe polyhydramnios, would you want to have your labour induced early to enable 'controlled' breaking of the waters, to plan a **caesarean** or to wait and see what position your baby is in and whether the head has engaged by the time your labour starts?

Also see "Baby's well-being – questions to ask", p.68.

Suspected poor growth

One of the main things that is checked at routine antenatal appointments is how well your baby is growing. This is because babies that are growing poorly seem to be at greater risk of **stillbirth**.

If a baby is not growing well in the womb it may be better for them to be born sooner, although depending how far along the pregnancy is, that will be a trade-off between the risks of continued poor growth in the womb and the risks of being born **prematurely**. Early birth could be by induction or a caesarean.

Not all babies that appear to be **SGA** (small for gestational age) have growth problems. It's estimated that 50–70% of them are naturally small (RCOG 2013c).

Given that induction may increase the stress a baby experiences during labour, it may not be helpful for a baby that is already vulnerable. The NICE Guideline on Induction (NICE 2008) does not recommend induction for babies with "**severe fetal growth restriction** and confirmed **fetal compromise**". In other words, it says labour should not be induced if a baby's growth is severely limited *and* tests have confirmed that the baby is not in good health.

The guidelines do not say anything about the situation where a baby's growth is only a little below average, or the baby is **SGA**, but there is no concern about their well-being. It is these babies that we consider here.

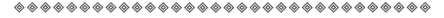

Research Evidence

The charts below show the findings of a recent study into stillbirths and SGA babies (Gardosi 2013). The definition of SGA used in the study was a predicted or actual birthweight below the 10th centile on a customised growth chart (known as a GROW chart). An example of a customised GROW chart can be seen here *www.perinatal.org. uk/growth/example.htm*.

The authors assume that the rate is lower when growth restriction was identified in pregnancy because those babies had an early birth, but the data does not show how many of the stillbirths occurred following induction or caesarean.

Stillbirths per 10,000 pregnancies

SGA babies detected or undetected in pregnancy vs whole population

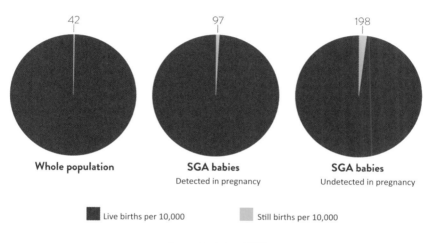

Source: Gardosi et al 2013

Just under 60% of the stillbirths of growth restricted babies occurred before 34 weeks, and around 70% before 37 weeks and there is no way of knowing whether these babies would have been saved by being born before that time. A planned **premature** birth might have increased their risk of **neonatal death**.

Another population study from Norway (Morken 2014) looked at **stillbirth** and **perinatal** death rates for SGA babies by week of pregnancy. The number of perinatal deaths *reduced* after 37 weeks, reaching a minimum at 40 weeks, and the stillbirth rate only began to rise substantially *after* 40 weeks. This suggests that it is only after 40 weeks that the benefit of elective birth in avoiding stillbirth may begin to outweigh the increase in neonatal deaths for SGA babies .

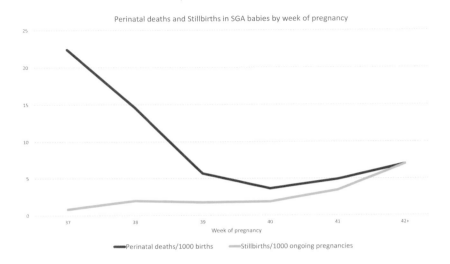

Perinatal deaths and Stillbirths in SGA babies by week of pregnancy

How Small for Gestational Age (SGA) babies are identified

The standard method is for a midwife to offer to measure the size of your bump at each antenatal appointment and to plot these on a **fetal growth chart** against the week of pregnancy. The chart shows the range of measurements that might be found at that point divided into 'centiles' (percentage bands), so that the 90th centile is the point below which 90% of the population would measure at that stage of pregnancy, and the 10th centile is the point below which only 10% would fall. By seeing which centile line the baby's growth appears to be following it is possible to predict the likely birthweight and see whether the growth appears to be at the expected rate.

If the measurements suggest that the baby's growth is below the 10th centile, or if the growth appears to be slowing, the midwife will probably recommend an ultrasound scan to check. People with other risk factors, such as being a smoker or having previously had an **SGA** baby, may be recommended to have regular ultrasound growth scans every 2–4 weeks throughout late pregnancy.

As discussed in *"Induction for predicted high birthweight" (p.52)*, ultrasound scans carried out in the third trimester can over- or underestimate the actual birthweight by as much as 10%.

Factors like your baby's sex and your height, weight, ethnic heritage, and how many pregnancies you have had all affect the natural size for your baby to be. Some NHS trusts have introduced customised GROW charts (as used in the Gardosi 2013 study above) which take account of these factors. It is thought that these should be more accurate at identifying SGA babies than the standard **growth charts**. If you are told that your baby is SGA it might be worth checking whether your midwife is using a customised GROW chart, especially if you are small yourself or if your ethnic heritage or family history makes it more likely that your babies will be small. An example of a computerised GROW chart can be seen here, *www.perinatal.org.uk/growth/example.htm*.

All of this is assuming that your baby's gestational age (the number of weeks of pregnancy) is known with certainty. An inaccurate estimated due date could lead to a baby being wrongly identified as SGA because they are younger than the due date suggests; or one who is older but is growth restricted being missed. For a discussion of the accuracy of estimated due dates, see *"How long a pregnancy is 'too long?", p.22* and the AIMS Birth Information web page, "How accurate is my due date?", *www.aims.org.uk/information/item/due-date*.

Does induction reduce the risk?

As mentioned above, the NICE guidelines (NICE 2008) say that induction **should not be done** if the baby appears to be in poor condition already, and the RCOG guidelines say that if a Doppler scan indicates a cause for concern a **caesarean** should be offered (RCOG 2013c).

If the baby is suspected to be SGA but there is no immediate concern, some consultants recommend early induction on the assumption that this will reduce the risk of a stillbirth.

In the study discussed above (Gardosi 2013), the authors assumed that the outcomes were better for SGA babies detected in pregnancy than for those that were only identified at birth because early detection allowed the birth to be brought forward. However, the Norwegian study suggests that induction before 40 weeks might have little effect on stillbirths but result in more **perinatal** deaths. At present, we do not have enough evidence to show whether it is always better to induce labour early when an SGA baby is suspected, or to continue the pregnancy with careful monitoring of the baby's well-being and only intervene if this gives cause for concern.

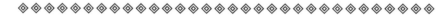

Research Evidence

There are only two small trials that looked directly at this question. The authors of the larger one (Boers 2010) say that "It is reasonable for patients who are keen on non-intervention to choose expectant management with intensive maternal and fetal monitoring because, as far as we can tell, this approach is safe for the baby." This same study also found that babies were less likely to be admitted to intensive care if they were born after 38 weeks, so "it is reasonable to delay [induction] until 38 weeks, provided [there is] watchful monitoring" (Boers 2010).

Induction for SGA babies seems to be associated with an increase in caesareans (RCOG 2013c). This may be because an already vulnerable baby cannot cope with the added stress of induction, and/or that early inductions are less likely to be successful.

How is the "Saving Babies' Lives Care Bundle" affecting outcomes for SGA babies?

In 2016 NHS England introduced a care bundle called "Saving Babies' Lives" (SBLCB)which aimed to reduce the national stillbirth rate. A care bundle is a package of measures which are expected to have an impact on a health issue, and one of the elements in this case is better identification of poorly-growing babies. Originally this meant all babies below the 10th centile.

An audit looking at data from before and after the introduction of the SBLCB in 19 NHS Trusts (Widdows 2018) found a reduction in stillbirths over this period, from around 4.1 out of every 1000 to 3.3 out of every 1000 births (so just under one fewer babies dying out of every 1000). The stillbirth rate in the UK was already decreasing before the SBLCB was introduced (Hickey 2019), and even the authors of the evaluation say only that "it is highly plausible that the SBLCB contributed to the fall in stillbirths" – they cannot be certain that it did so (Widdows 2018). It's also not possible to say how much the detection of SGA babies might have contributed to any reduction compared to the other three elements of the bundle.

The introduction of the care bundle has resulted in many more interventions including more ultrasound scans, inductions and unplanned caesareans. The report highlights this risk of 'intervention creep' and stresses the need to better target interventions. It also cautions against induction before 39 weeks unless there is evidence that the baby's well-being is being compromised, because birth before 39 weeks carries health risks for the baby.

Interestingly, the audit also found that there were more pre-term births and more babies admitted to a neonatal intensive care unit following introduction of the care bundle.

As a result the latest version focuses on babies under the 3rd centile or with other risk factors. It recommends that birth "should occur" at 37+0 and no later than 37+6 weeks for babies under the 3rd centile and be offered at 39 weeks for those between the 3rd and 10th centile, provided there is no other cause for concern.

» » »» » »» » »» » »» » »» » »» » »» » »» » » » »» » » »

Summary

- » The majority of babies who are SGA are born in good health, and many of these will be naturally small rather than suffering restricted growth.

- » Detecting that a baby is growing poorly during pregnancy seems to reduce the risk of stillbirth, but if an induction or caesarean is done too early that may increase the chances of a baby suffering poor health or even dying soon after birth.

» At present, we do not have enough evidence to show whether it is always better to induce labour early when an SGA baby is suspected, or to continue the pregnancy with careful monitoring of the baby's well-being and only intervene if this gives cause for concern.

» Induction for SGA babies seems to be associated with an increase in caesareans (RCOG 2013c).

Things to consider

- Are your midwife and doctor using a **GROW chart** which has been customised to take account of things like your height, weight and ethnic heritage?
- Do you think the estimated due date is correct?
- How severe does the growth restriction seem to be? If it is borderline, you might want to have another ultrasound scan to check before you make any decision.
- Does your baby appear to be well otherwise?
- If your baby is thought to be SGA but otherwise well, would you rather have your labour induced, plan a caesarean or wait to go into labour unless a problem with her/his well-being is detected later?

Also see "Baby's well-being – questions to ask", p.68.

Health problems in pregnancy

Sometimes health problems develop during pregnancy which can only be resolved by the birth of the baby. These include Intrahepatic Cholestasis of Pregnancy (ICP) (also known as obstetric cholestasis), high blood pressure and **pre-eclampsia.**

Depending on how severe the problem is, these may pose health risks for you, your baby or both. Sometimes the problem can worsen suddenly and unpredictably. If you are affected by one of these problems, **make sure your midwife or doctor tells you the warning signs.**

How might this affect the timing of the birth?

If you develop a serious health problem during pregnancy your midwife or doctor may recommend an early birth by induction or caesarean. The current recommendations about the timing of for the most common problems are discussed below.

As discussed in *"Deciding about induction before 39 weeks", p.13,* early birth carries some risks, especially for **premature** babies. Even **early term** babies (born between 37 and 39 weeks) are more likely to experience health problems including breathing difficulties than those born after 39 weeks (ACOG 2013), so if the problem is not severe and does not worsen, some people will choose to wait at least till 37 or till 39 weeks.

Your decision about whether to bring the birth forward, and whether to have induction or a planned caesarean, may therefore depend on how many weeks pregnant you are, the current health of you and your baby and how severe the problem seems to be. **It's important to get clear information on these points from your doctors and midwives.**

Questions to ask

You need to be given information about *your specific situation* to enable you to weigh up the risks and benefits of the different options. The kind of things you might want to be informed about include:

- How certain is the diagnosis? (If it is border-line it might be worth asking to be retested before making any decision.)
- How serious does the problem seem to be?
- What warning signs might mean that the condition is worsening?
- What are the possible risks to me and my baby of continuing the pregnancy, at least up to a certain point (e.g. to 37 or 39 weeks)? How would our well-being be monitored during this time?

- If my baby was born **prematurely** or at **early term**, what are the possible risks or other consequences of that? What care might be needed once they were born?
- What are the risks, benefits and likelihood of success of induction in this situation, at this stage of pregnancy?
- What are the risks and benefits of a **caesarean** for me and my baby?

Each of the three most common problems is discussed in detail below.

Intrahepatic Cholestasis (ICP)/(Obstetric Cholestasis)

ICP (formerly known as obstetric cholestasis) occurs when bile acids (produced in the liver to help with fat absorption) build up in the bloodstream. It is thought to affect about seven in every 1000 pregnant women a year in the UK but most of these cases are mild.

The main symptom is itching with no rash, which, though it can be distressing, is not dangerous, but very high levels of bile acids can harm the baby and may even cause stillbirth.

Itching in pregnancy can happen for other reasons so doesn't necessarily mean you have ICP but is always worth discussing with your midwife. If it continues, or if you have other symptoms like dark urine, pale bowel movements and/or pain around your liver, you should be offered a blood test to check.

If you are diagnosed with ICP, or if you are not diagnosed but the itching continues **make sure you are offered regular tests** to monitor the level of bile acids in your blood, in case the levels rise. (*See "What monitoring is recommended?", p.86.*)

The current RCOG guidelines (RCOG 2011b) suggest induction after 37 weeks if ICP is diagnosed but admit that this is not evidence based. Research published since then suggests that may only be necessary if the ICP is very severe (Ovadia 2019).

There haven't been any trials comparing induction with **expectant management** when ICP has been diagnosed.

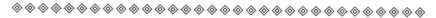

Research Evidence

A review of the available evidence (Ovadia 2019) found that the risk of stillbirth is only increased when the serum bile acids concentration is 100 μmol/L (100 micromoles per litre) or more. Out of every 100 mothers with this level three or four would have a stillbirth and 96–97 would not. At this serum bile acid level the risk of stillbirth was higher throughout pregnancy. It appeared to increase with the length of pregnancy, but more rapidly after 36 weeks.

Most people with ICP have levels lower than 100 μmol/L, and their risk of stillbirth was found to be no higher than for those who do not have ICP (see table below). The authors concluded that if the serum bile acid concentration is under 100 μmol/L, people "can probably be reassured that the risk of stillbirth is similar to that of pregnant women in the general population, provided repeat bile acid testing is done until delivery."

	Stillbirth risk	
National average (2015)	0.33%	
ICP with serum bile acids below 40 μmol/L	0.13%	
ICP with serum bile acids between 40 and 99 μmol/L	0.28%	
ICP with serum bile acids of 100 μmol/L or more	3.44%	

A **population study** (Geenes 2014) found that 70% of the stillbirths in their sample of mothers with ICP were to women who had other pregnancy complications (such as **pre-eclampsia** and gestational diabetes) in addition to ICP. They suggest that these women need closer monitoring than those with ICP alone.

What monitoring is recommended?

The latest research has not yet been incorporated into official guidelines, but the organisation ICP support (*www.icpsupport.org*) has suggested the following:

- Itching persists, bile acids and liver function tests are normal:
  » Test every 2–3 weeks till 34 weeks, then weekly.

- Itching persists, bile acids are normal, liver function tests are not:
  - » Check for other causes of liver problems.
  - » Test every two weeks till 34 weeks, then weekly.

- Bile acids are raised:
  - » Check for other causes of liver problems; if negative consider drug treatment for ICP.
  - » Test twice-weekly.

» » »» » »» » »» » »» » »» » »» » »» » »» » »» » »» » » » »» » » »

Summary

- » If you have ICP but your serum bile acids concentration is below 100 µmol/L (100 micromoles per litre) your risk of a stillbirth appears to be no higher than for the general population.
- » There seems to be no evidence to support a need for pre-term or **early term birth** if your level remains below 100umol/L **but you should be offered regular tests to check for any rise.**
- » If your serum bile acid level is 100 umol/L or more there is an increased risk of stillbirth though 96–97 out of 100 women with this level will not suffer one.
- » The risk for this group seems to rise more steeply after about 36 weeks. Birth before 36 weeks may reduce the risk, though there is no way to predict which babies will be affected.

See also "Health problems in pregnancy – Questions to ask", p.84.

High blood pressure

Having high blood pressure before becoming pregnant is called **chronic hypertension** and high blood pressure developing during pregnancy is called **gestational hypertension**.

If you have chronic hypertension NICE recommends that when planning your pregnancy you should be offered a discussion of the risks and benefits of treatment with a specialist in hypertensive disorders of pregnancy. Once pregnant you should be offered weekly antenatal appointments if your hypertension is poorly controlled and appointments every two to four weeks if it is well-controlled. (NICE 2019)

If you develop gestational hypertension you should be offered a full assessment by a healthcare professional who is trained in the management of hypertensive disorders of pregnancy when the problem is identified. (NICE 2019).

How might this affect the timing of birth?

If you have either chronic hypertension (whether or not it is being controlled with drugs) or gestational hypertension NICE recommends that as long as your blood pressure reading is under 160/110, you should *not* be offered planned early birth before 37 weeks.

After 37 weeks, if your blood pressure remains under 160/110 you should have an opportunity to discuss the timing of the birth, and any other factors that might affect that, with a senior obstetrician. (Remember that the decision about whether to plan an induction or caesarean or wait for labour to start is yours.)

If your blood pressure cannot be controlled below 160/110 and/or you have any other warning signs you should be offered admission to hospital for further tests and monitoring for **pre-eclampsia** (see below).

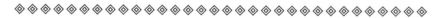

Research Evidence

There seems to be no evidence to support induction or caesarean after 37 weeks for those with hypertension unless their blood pressure becomes raised to a dangerous level, they develop pre-eclampsia, or there are other concerns about the baby's well-being.

The NICE **GDG** found only one small study about chronic hypertension (Hamed 2014), and one about gestational hypertension (Koopmans 2009). These were both far too small to detect any difference in stillbirths rates and found no difference in outcomes for mothers with mild to moderate hypertension.

Someone with chronic hypertension is more likely to have an underlying problem with their blood circulation and so are more likely to have babies that are growth restricted. It is this that may affect the timing of the birth rather than their blood pressure as such *(see "Induction for suspected poor growth", p.76)*

» » »» » »»» » »»» » »»» » »»» » »»» » »»» » »»» » »»» » » » »»» » » »

Summary

> » If your blood pressure is lower than 160/110mmHg induction is not recommended before 37 weeks unless there are other reasons for it.
> » If your blood pressure remains lower than 160/110mmHg after 37 weeks you should have a chance to discuss the timing of birth with a senior doctor.
> » There is no evidence that early birth has any benefit when mild to moderate hypertension is the only problem.
> » If your blood pressure remains over 160/110mmHg even after treatment you should be offered further tests and monitoring for **pre-eclampsia** (see below).

See also "Health problems in pregnancy – Questions to ask", p.84.

Pre-eclampsia

Pre-eclampsia is a condition that can develop in the second half of pregnancy (and occasionally earlier or after the birth). Mild pre-eclampsia affects up to 6% of pregnancies and usually causes no problems, but it is potentially very serious – and sometimes even life-threatening – for both mother and baby. Only 1-2% of mothers have it severely, but mild cases can become more severe very suddenly and unpredictably. Rarely (about one in 4000 pregnancies), it can progress to eclampsia (fits), which can cause brain damage or even the death of a mother, or cause a baby to be stillborn. **Make sure** your midwife tells you the warning signs that pre-eclampsia is becoming more severe and seek immediate help if you think it is happening. There is also information on the signs to watch out for here: *www.nhs.uk/conditions/pre-eclampsia/symptoms/*.

The first signs of pre-eclampsia are usually picked up at a routine antenatal appointment through checks for high blood pressure and protein in the urine.

How might this affect the timing of birth?

The only cure is for the baby to be born, so this may mean the baby needs to be born **prematurely**, and if the situation is urgent a **caesarean** may be required.

NICE guidelines on Hypertension in pregnancy (NICE 2019) make different recommendations according to when pre-eclampsia is diagnosed:

Before 37 weeks:

- Continue regular monitoring unless there is a cause for concern that outweighs the risks of premature birth.
- When considering the option of planned early birth, take into account the woman's and baby's condition, risk factors and availability of neonatal unit beds.

From Week 37 onwards

- Recommend birth within 24–48 hours.

Depending on the circumstances and how quickly your baby needs to be born, as well as your own preferences, you might choose a caesarean or induction of labour.

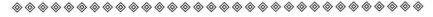

Research Evidence

There have been several small studies which found that if severe pre-eclampsia occurs before 34 weeks, **expectant management** (waiting for labour) seemed to cause fewer health problems for the babies than immediate induction did, but the evidence isn't good enough to show which is better for the mother's health (Churchill 2018).

For pre-eclampsia which develops after 34 weeks the NICE guidelines say that "There was limited evidence on the benefits and harms of **planned early birth** compared with **expectant management** of pregnancy". However, based on the one randomised controlled trial (the HYPITAT-II study, Broekhuijsen 2015) which was available at the time they decided that these pregnancies "could be managed with continued surveillance to 37 weeks, unless there were specific concerns or indications to offer a planned early birth before then".

The HYPITAT II study was of mothers with "non-severe hypertensive disorders". It found that immediate birth between 34 and 37 weeks of pregnancy reduced the number of mothers who developed more severe problems (from 3.1% in the expectant management group to 1.1%) but increased the number of babies with severe breathing problems (from 1.7% to 5.7%). However, many of the mothers included in this trial did not have pre-eclampsia.

A UK-based trial has been published since which looked only at mothers who developed pre-eclampsia between 34 and 37 weeks (the Phoenix trial, Chappell 2019). This found that when labour was induced within two days of pre-eclampsia being diagnosed fewer mothers suffered serious health problems (15% in the **early birth** group vs 20% in the expectant management group – so five fewer women per 100), had severely raised blood pressure (60% vs 69% – nine fewer women per 100) or progressed to severe pre-eclampsia (64% vs 74% – ten fewer women per 100).

Over half the mothers assigned to the expectant management group actually "had medically indicated delivery before 37 weeks."

None of the babies in either group were stillborn or suffered a **neonatal death**. Significantly more in the early birth group were admitted to a neonatal unit (42% vs 34% – eight more per 100), though the main reason for admission was prematurity and in contrast to the HYPITAT-II study the numbers having serious breathing problems were similar in the two groups.

The authors conclude "our trial supports offering induction to women with late preterm pre-eclampsia" though the trade-off of fewer serious health problems for mothers against higher neonatal unit admissions "should be discussed with women with late preterm pre-eclampsia to allow shared decision making on timing of delivery."

» » »» » »» » »» » »» » »» » »» » »» » »» » »» » » » »» » » »

Summary

» Pre-eclampsia is usually a mild condition, but it is potentially serious. The condition can worsen very suddenly and require immediate action. In some cases, this could mean an immediate **caesarean**.

» The timing of birth if you develop pre-eclampsia needs to balance of the risks of **premature** birth versus the risks of continuing the pregnancy.

» There is some evidence that if severe pre-eclampsia develops before 34 weeks it is better for the baby's health to delay the birth, but we don't know what effect this has on outcomes for the mother.

» Currently NICE recommends continuing the pregnancy till 37 weeks if possible, but there is now evidence that birth within two days of diagnosis is better for mothers who develop severe pre-eclampsia after 34 weeks but may result in more babies being admitted to a neonatal unit.

See also "Questions to ask", p.84.

IVF pregnancy

Pregnant women and people who conceived using IVF (in vitro fertilisation) are often told that their pregnancy should not go beyond a certain point (typically 40 weeks) because they have an increased risk of stillbirth. However, this seems to be a recent practice because it is not one of the reasons for induction listed in the NICE Guidelines on inducing labour (NICE 2008).

Though the risk of stillbirth appears to be a bit higher in IVF than in non-IVF pregnancies, the absolute risk is low.

There is often a concern that people who need IVF to get pregnant are likely to be older than average. The issue of age is considered in *"Your age" p.45,* so in this section we will only consider the evidence around induction because of IVF.

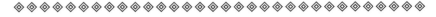

Research Evidence

There appears to be an increase in the risk of **perinatal** death for babies conceived through IVF, but different studies produce different results for how much greater this risk is (RCOG 2012). This is probably because in small studies the results are affected by random variations .

Studies also varied in how early in pregnancy they started to record outcomes. Some included women from 16 weeks of pregnancy, others from 28 weeks. This could make a big difference to the findings if a high proportion of the perinatal deaths in IVF pregnancies occur with births that happen early in pregnancy.

One review (Helmerhorst 2004) which combined the results of 9 studies suggested that perinatal death is around 1.7 times more common in single babies conceived by IVF compared to those conceived spontaneously. The absolute risk was around twelve babies in every 1000 IVF pregnancies (so 988 survived), and eight in every 1000 non-IVF pregnancies (so 992 survived). For comparison, the overall perinatal death rate in the UK is about six in every thousand births overall and nine in every thousand births to mothers aged over 40 (MBRRACE 2016).

Interestingly, most of the studies in this review found a *lower* risk of perinatal death for twins conceived by IVF (roughly 20 in every 1000 pregnancies) than for twins conceived spontaneously (around 40 in every 1000 pregnancies). This may be because they are less likely to be identical.

Another, larger review of perinatal death rates (Qin 2016) included 22 studies and found that perinatal deaths were around 1.6 times more common in IVF pregnancies. Unfortunately, it does not include data on the absolute risk, or the timing of the births.

These studies all suggest that the risk of perinatal death is a bit higher overall for IVF pregnancies, but the absolute risk remains small. What is not clear is how the risk changes as pregnancy progresses. One study carried out in the Nordic countries (Henningsen et al 2016) suggests that the increase in stillbirth rates may only apply to babies conceived by IVF who are born at under 28 weeks of pregnancy, and that there is no significant difference for those born later.

It is known that IVF pregnancies are associated with a higher chance of there being health complications for mother or baby (RCOG 2012) which can affect the chances of stillbirth or **neonatal death**. Healthy mothers who conceived by IVF could potentially have a lower risk of perinatal death than those with a health problem, but unfortunately no studies seem to have looked at this.

Does induction reduce the risk?

The short answer is no one knows. The research simply hasn't been done, and the Royal College of Obstetricians and Gynaecologists has stated as much "There is no evidence to show whether early labour induction improves outcomes for IVF babies." (RCOG Query bank reply 2013b)

How accurate is the estimated due date for IVF babies?

If you conceived by IVF you will know, to within a couple of days, when the fertilised egg implanted in your womb, based on the date of the embryo transfer process. With this information, you should be able to estimate a due date for the baby.

One study on length of non-IVF pregnancy (Jukic 2013) found that labour starts on average 259 days (37 weeks) after the egg implants in the womb. So if you add 37 weeks to the date of your embryo transfer procedure that should give you a reasonable estimate of a due date to compare with any ultrasound estimate that you are given.

A recent study (Knight 2018) found that for women who conceived by IVF, and therefore knew when their egg was fertilised, the routine ultrasound dating scan consistently put their estimated birth date earlier than it should have been by an average of three days.

Despite this, we sometimes hear of midwives or doctors using a date estimated from ultrasound to recommend the timing of birth even if this doesn't seem to agree with the date the egg was fertilised.

The AIMS Birth Information web page "How accurate is my due date?", *www.aims.org.uk/information/item/due-date* explains the uncertainties around the estimation of due dates, including for IVF babies.

» » »» » »» » »» » »» » »» » »» » »» » »» » »» » » » »» » » »

Summary

» Due to the limited evidence we can't be sure, but it's possible that if the mother is healthy, the pregnancy has been straightforward and the baby is growing normally, then a baby conceived by IVF may be at no greater risk than one conceived spontaneously once the pregnancy has gone beyond 28 weeks.

» The risk of a **perinatal** death appears to be 60-70% higher for a single baby conceived by IVF compared to non-IVF pregnancies but the absolute risk is still low. Estimates vary but probably around 12 IVF babies in every 1000 suffer a perinatal death, and the majority (988) will survive birth.

» The higher risk may be partly due to mothers who have had IVF being at greater risk of health problems which could affect their baby's well-being.

» It is also possible that the increased risk only exists because of a higher rate of stillbirths before 28 weeks of pregnancy amongst babies conceived by IVF, and that in late pregnancy the risk is no different from that of other babies.

» There is evidence that the risk for twins conceived by IVF is lower than for non-IVF twins.

» There is no evidence *at all* to show whether it is better to induce labour if birth has not occurred by 40 weeks of pregnancy, simply because the baby was conceived by IVF.

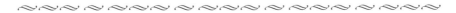

Things to consider

- Are you carrying more than one baby? Considerations for twins or higher multiples will be different from those for single babies.
- Are you healthy and has your pregnancy been straightforward up to this point?
- Are there any reasons for concern about your baby's well-being other than that they were conceived with IVF?

- How do you feel about the possible risks of a medical induction and the possibility of needing an unplanned **caesarean** if it fails?
- Does the estimated due date in your notes make sense compared with the time at which the egg was fertilised?

VBAC labour

This section only considers the potential impact of induction on VBAC success and risks. For more information on VBAC generally see the AIMS book, "Birth after Caesarean".

Induction might be recommended to someone planning a VBAC for any of the reasons discussed in this book. The considerations will be the same as for anyone, but with the addition of concerns over the impact of induction on the chances of a successful VBAC and the risk of uterine rupture, which is when the scar on the womb left by one or more previous caesareans separates.

Because of these concerns, the RCOG guideline says that a decision about inducing or augmenting a VBAC labour needs careful consideration and you should be able to discuss it with a senior obstetrician (RCOG 2015). This should include discussion of the method of induction and whether to use **oxytocin** to speed the labour up. (For an explanation of the methods discussed in this section see *"Methods of Medical Induction", p.108.*)

Though the risks in a VBAC labour are increased by induction or **augmentation** they remain low.

A recent NICE guideline (NICE 2019b) includes the following:

"When discussing oxytocin for delay in the first or second stage of labour, explain to women who have had a previous caesarean section that this:

» increases the chance of uterine rupture
» reduces the chance of another caesarean section
» increases the chance of an instrumental birth."

Note that for all these points the evidence was described as being "very low quality".

NICE also advises *against* routinely offering to break the waters in a VBAC labour as there isn't any evidence to support the practice (NICE 2019b).

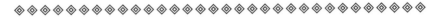

Research Evidence

Different studies vary quite a lot in the rates that they report but overall it seems that induction reduces the chances of a successful VBAC from around 75-80% to around 65% (Landon 2004, Guise 2010).

The absolute risk of uterine rupture is very low in all circumstances, but it does appear to be slightly higher when the labour is induced, or when it is augmented with synthetic **oxytocin**. The scale of the risk seems to depend on the methods used. In the most recent UK study (the UKOSS study, Fitzpatrick 2012) just over one out of every 1000 women whose VBAC labour started spontaneously, experienced a rupture, compared with three out of every 1000 women who had a VBAC labour induced with prostaglandin and/or had an oxytocin drip in labour. The figure was slightly higher for those that used prostaglandin to start the labour, with or without subsequent use of oxytocin (3.6/1000) than for those that had synthetic oxytocin alone (2.8/1000).

This may be because prostaglandin works at least in part by stimulating the production of an enzyme which breaks down a substance in the cervix called collagen (Buhimschi, 2005). Collagen is present in scar tissue so prostaglandin may weaken the scar.

There is evidence that using a Foley catheter can be as effective as prostaglandin in inducing labour, with less risk of overstimulating the muscles of the womb and no difference in unplanned caesareans (Jozwiak 2012) but the studies on which this was based did not distinguish between mothers who had or had not had a previous caesarean and did not comment on the risk of uterine rupture with this method.

There is some low-quality evidence from **population studies** that mechanical methods of induction may be safer for VBAC labours. One large US study (Landon 2004) found that the risk of uterine rupture for women who had induction with prostaglandin was fourteen out of 1000, compared to about four out of 1000 for those who went into labour spontaneously. For those that had their labours induced by mechanical dilation methods with or without an oxytocin drip the risk was nine out of 1000. (Note that this is an older US study which may be why the figures for all groups are higher than found in the UKOSS study discussed above).

A couple of studies looking at the dose of synthetic oxytocin used for augmentation found (not surprisingly) that the risk rises as the dose is increased (Cahill 2007, Cahill 2008). *See "What are the benefits and risks of synthetic oxytocin?" p, 122.*

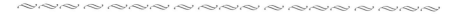

Summary

» Induction reduces the chance of a successful VBAC but around two-thirds of mothers planning a VBAC will give birth vaginally following induction.

» Induction slightly increases the chances of the scar on the womb opening, but this remains rare (about 3 in every 1000 induced VBAC labours).

» A mechanical method of induction may be safer than **prostaglandin** for induction of a VBAC labour, but the evidence for this is limited.

Things to consider

• How do you feel about the possible impact of induction on your chances of a successful VBAC and the increase in the chances of a uterine rupture compared with if you waited for your labour to start?

• For what reason are you being recommended to have your labour induced? How good is the evidence for this recommendation and how do you feel about it?

• If you choose induction, would you prefer to try a mechanical method rather than **prostaglandin**?

• If your baby needs to be born early, would you prefer a planned caesarean to an induced VBAC labour?

• How would you feel about the increased chances of a uterine rupture if you were to have an **oxytocin** drip to speed up your labour versus the possibly lower chance of having a repeat caesarean?

Twins and triplets

There are many issues to do with the birth of twins and triplets which are outside the scope of this book. Here we will only consider the evidence around timing of birth and the choice of induction method.

For many people carrying more than one baby, the question of induction will not arise because for about 60% of twin pregnancies spontaneous labour starts before 37 weeks and in about 75% of triplets pregnancies it starts by 35 weeks (NICE 2019c).

The timing of birth for twins or triplets is a trade-off between the possible increase in the chances of a **stillbirth** if the pregnancy continues, and the possible increase in the risk of a **neonatal death** due to prematurity or low birth weight, as twins are usually lower in birthweight than single babies of the same age.

The NICE guideline (2019c), "Twin and triplet pregnancy" has different recommendations for the timing of planned birth for the different types of twin and triplet pregnancy. For definitions of the terms describing these see the glossary and this article *www.aims.org.uk/journal/item/multiple-multiples*. If you are not sure which applies to your babies, ask your midwife or doctor.

- Offer planned birth at 37 weeks for an uncomplicated dichorionic diamniotic (DCDA) twin pregnancy.
- Offer planned birth after a course of antenatal corticosteroids has been considered:
  - » at 36 weeks for uncomplicated MCDA (monochorionic diamniotic) twin pregnancy
  - » between 32+0 and 33+6 weeks for uncomplicated MCMA (monochorionic monoamniotic) twin pregnancy
  - » at 35 weeks for TCTA (trichorionic triamniotic) or DCTA (dichorionic triamniotic) triplet pregnancy.

For more complicated cases NICE suggests an individual assessment.

If you decline planned birth at the recommended time, you should be offered weekly appointments with a specialist obstetrician, with "an ultrasound scan and assessment of amniotic fluid level and doppler of the umbilical artery flow for each baby, in addition to fortnightly fetal growth scans." This makes it clear that it is your decision whether to accept a planned birth at the recommended time.

All these recommendations assume that the estimated due date is accurate. (See the AIMS Birth Information web page "How accurate is my due date?", *www.aims.org.uk/information/item/due-date*.)

The guidelines do not make any recommendation about whether a planned birth should be by induction or caesarean (which may depend on the positions of the babies), nor what method of induction should be used.

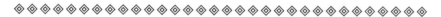

Research Evidence

As twins are relatively uncommon, and triplets even more so, it would be almost impossible to conduct a randomised controlled trial to determine what impact a **planned early birth** has on the number of **perinatal** deaths.

In fact the **GDG** say, "There was not enough good evidence to conclusively identify the optimal timing of birth according to chorionicity and amnionicity, so the committee also used their expertise and experience to make recommendations." They mainly based their recommendations on the pooled results of 10 **population studies** of different types of twins but found no useful evidence about triplets. Unfortunately they do not state in their analysis what the absolute risks are by week of pregnancy – just at what point risks seem to increase or decrease.

The best evidence we have therefore comes from a review of population studies that looked at the rates of stillbirth and **neonatal death** for twins born at each week of pregnancy (Cheong-See 2016).

This review does not distinguish between the type of labour (spontaneous or induced) and birth (vaginal or caesarean) nor between mothers with or without health issues, meaning we can't be sure how the increase in risk might vary for these different groups.

Dichorionic (DCDA) twins

The Cheong-See (2016) review suggests that for uncomplicated dichorionic twin pregnancies the risk of stillbirth rises and the risk of **neonatal death** falls as pregnancy continues so that the risk of perinatal death is lowest between 37 and 38 weeks of pregnancy. At this point the stillbirth rate was 3.4 per 1000 ongoing pregnancies and the neonatal death rate 2.2 per 1000 births.

After 38 weeks the rise in the risk of stillbirth started to outweigh the fall in neonatal deaths. The stillbirth rate for dichorionic twins born after 38 weeks was 10.6 per 1000 ongoing pregnancies and the neonatal death rate was 1.5 per 1000 births. There were not enough births beyond 39 weeks to measure the risk of waiting longer.

Monochorionic (MCDA & MCMA) twins

The **perinatal** death rate for uncomplicated monochorionic twin pregnancies appeared to be higher than for dichorionic twins at all weeks of pregnancy but there is no good evidence about the best time for them to be born. The review (Cheong-See 2016) was unable to detect a significant difference in risk between birth at 36, 37 or 38 weeks. It did not look separately at MCDA and MCMA twins, but for all monochorionic twins at 37 weeks the stillbirth rate was 9.6 per 1000, and the **neonatal death** rate 3.6 per 1000.

The pooled results of the population studies used by the **GDG** seemed to suggest a possible increase in stillbirths beyond 36 weeks for MCDA twins, so though the evidence is not strong they decided to recommend planned birth at 36 weeks. This is "to reflect the higher risk and complexity of this type of pregnancy" and the fact that birth at this point did not appear to be linked to an increase in neonatal deaths or serious health problems (NICE 2019c).

The GDG found two studies of MCMA twins, which showed the risk of neonatal death to be at its lowest at 34 weeks. Based on this plus their "own knowledge and experience" they decided to recommend offering planned birth between 32+0 and 33+6 weeks for MCMA twins. Note that babies born this early are very likely to need to spend time in a neonatal unit.

Triplets

For triplets the evidence is very limited, but some studies indicate that the risk may be at its lowest at 34–36 weeks, hence the NICE recommendation to offer planned early birth at 35 weeks.

How should labour be induced in twin pregnancies?

There are only a couple of studies that have compared different methods of induction for mothers carrying twins (and none for triplets) and, unfortunately, they produced slightly different results.

A **population study** in Sweden (Jonsson 2015) found that 79% of the mothers of twins who had their labours induced had a vaginal birth, compared to 88% of those who went into labour spontaneously. The chance of having a **caesarean** appeared to be significantly higher if the mother had either **prostaglandin** or a Foley catheter to encourage cervical ripening (37%) or had an **oxytocin** drip (36%) than if she only had her waters broken (15%). That may be misleading, as it is not possible to break the waters unless a mother's cervix has already begun to dilate. So that group were presumably already in early labour and would be less likely to have a failed induction than those needing a cervical ripening method.

Further analysis of the data collected for the Twin Birth Study (Mei-Dan 2017, which compared planned caesarean and planned vaginal birth outcomes for twins) found that 40% of those who had an induction had an unplanned caesarean, regardless of whether prostaglandin, **ARM** or an oxytocin drip were used.

It therefore seems that in twin pregnancies, unless the cervix is already starting to dilate, there is an unplanned caesarean rate of 35-40% with any method of induction.

» » »» » »» » »» » »» » »» » »» » »» » »» » »» » »» » » » »» » » »

Summary

» Many mothers with multiple pregnancies will go into spontaneous labour before the question of planned early birth arises.

» There isn't any direct evidence to show whether **planned early birth** or **expectant management** is generally better for multiple pregnancies.

» The current recommendations are for planned birth at 37 weeks for DCDA twins and at 36 weeks for MCDA twins if there are no other complications. These timings are based on the **population studies** discussed in the evidence section above. These studies cannot tell us whether the risks might be affected by other factors, such as whether the babies were born after spontaneous labour, induction or by caesarean or whether there were any pregnancy complications.

» There is limited evidence that the risk of **perinatal death** rises slightly beyond 37 weeks for DCDA twins and possibly rises beyond 36 weeks for MCDA twins. However most twins born later than this survive if there are no other complications.

» There is very little evidence to show when it is best for MCMA twins or for triplets to be born but current guidelines suggest between 32 and 34 weeks, and at 35 weeks respectively.

» Mothers carrying twins who have their labours induced appear to have a 35-40% chance of an unplanned caesarean.

Things to consider

- Is your preference for vaginal birth or **caesarean**?
- How do you feel about the increase in the risk of stillbirth if you waited a while longer to see if your labour would start spontaneously?
- How do you feel about the possible risks of a medical induction and the possibility of needing an unplanned caesarean if it fails?
- Do you think the estimated due date in your notes is accurate?
- If your babies were conceived by IVF, does the estimated due date make sense compared with the time at which the IVF was done? *(See "How accurate is the estimated due date for IVF babies?", p.94.)*

~~~~~

Chapter 3

Induction of labour

Spontaneous labour

Spontaneous labour is labour that starts without any artificial assistance.

No one is sure what exactly brings on labour, and there are probably several factors involved, but there is increasing evidence that the baby sends chemical signals when they are ready to be born (Gao 2015), and in particular when their lungs are ready to start breathing. This causes the release of chemicals called **prostaglandins** which bring about the ripening of the cervix.

During pregnancy, the cervix (the ring of muscles at the bottom of the womb) is keeping the baby safe inside, so it is usually closed, long and firm, and points slightly towards the back. As your body gets ready for labour, the muscle fibres in the cervix become softer and then begin to be drawn up, causing the cervix to become thinner and move forwards. This process is called 'ripening' of the cervix and often happens before any labour contractions.

Labour contractions are brought on and sustained by a hormone called **oxytocin** which is produced in the brain and then travels through the bloodstream to the muscles of the womb causing them to contract (shorten). When the womb muscles contract, they draw the now softened cervix upwards, causing it to open gradually. This is called dilation.

Ripening/dilation of the cervix

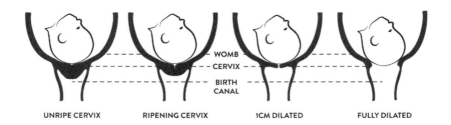

UNRIPE CERVIX   RIPENING CERVIX   1CM DILATED   FULLY DILATED

You may hear different terms used to describe the stages of labour.

First stage is usually defined as the period from when the cervix begins to dilate until it has opened enough for the baby's head to pass through – a diameter of roughly 10cm. It can be more useful to think of this as a 2-step process.

Early first stage (sometimes called the latent phase of labour) is defined by the NICE guideline on Intrapartum Care (NICE 2017) as the time from when the labour contractions start until the cervix has dilated up to 4cm. It's not uncommon for the contractions to start and stop repeatedly during this time, and it can last several days, especially with a first baby.

Active (or established) labour is the period when there are regular powerful contractions and the cervix is progressively dilating from 4cm to about 10cm. On average this lasts eight hours for a first baby and is rarely longer than 18 hours. If you have had a baby before, the average is five hours and it's rarely more than 12 hours.

The *second stage* is when you are pushing your baby down the birth canal. It ends when your baby is born. (NICE 2017)

Signs that your body is preparing for labour

There are many physical and emotional changes which indicate this. These could include:

»   Braxton-Hicks contractions (the 'practice' contractions which you may experience during pregnancy) becoming stronger.

»   Your baby's head engaging (moving down into your pelvis). You may notice that you've started to waddle!

»   Mild diarrhoea and/or vomiting. These are quite common in the last day or two before the birth but if severe or prolonged, or you have a fever, seek medical advice.

»   Having a 'show' (the appearance of the plug of jelly-like mucus that has been filling the gap in your cervix). This can happen up to two weeks before your labour begins.

»   A 'nesting instinct' – an urge to prepare for the arrival of your baby.

»   An instinctive awareness of changes in your body.

»   Yours waters breaking (though this only occurs before the start of contractions in about 10% of labours.)

You can also ask your midwife or doctor to assess something called the **Bishop's score** which is an estimate of how close your labour is to starting, based on how far your baby has moved down into your pelvis and the progress of the changes in your cervix. *(See "What is the Bishop's score and why is it important?", p.109.)*

What is induction of labour?

All methods of induction are trying to stimulate and mimic spontaneous labour. The term induction is usually applied to the use of medical methods, but there are also non-medical alternatives that you might like to try to encourage your labour to start.

Non-medical methods of induction

If you are keen to avoid medical induction but want to try to encourage your labour to start you may decide to try self-help methods or complementary therapies. Using these non-medical methods may help you to feel more in control and more able to relax, which could in itself make it more likely that your labour will begin without the need for medical induction.

Unfortunately, very little research has been done on the effectiveness or safety of these methods and most of the studies that have been done were small, but here is a summary of what is currently known.

Nipple stimulation

There is evidence (Kavanagh 2005) that nipple stimulation can make a significant difference to the chances of going into labour within 72 hours, though possibly only if the cervix has already begun to ripen. It also seems to reduce the chances of serious blood loss after birth. This is assumed to be because nipple stimulation encourages the production of **oxytocin.**

Acupuncture

There is some very limited evidence that acupuncture (using special needles to stimulate certain points on the body) or acupressure (applying pressure to these points) may help to ripen the cervix and therefore encourage labour to start (Smith 2017). These techniques have been used in China probably for thousands of years.

Homeopathy, reflexology, or hypnotherapy

There isn't enough evidence from **randomised controlled trials** to show whether other approaches like homeopathy, reflexology, or hypnotherapy are effective, but many people say that they have used these successfully and as far as we know there are unlikely to be any side effects.

Aromatherapy

Again there is little evidence, but it may be helpful. Some essential oils are not advised for use in pregnancy as they can be toxic to the unborn baby, so check with a qualified person which ones are safe to try.

Other methods

You may hear about other methods which have been used to bring on labour such as castor oil, pineapple, curry, sex and more. Unfortunately, we do not have enough research evidence to show whether these are effective.

Methods of medical induction

There are two phases to a medical induction: first there are interventions to ripen the cervix and encourage labour to start, and then intervention to strengthen or start contractions if necessary. Practices vary between hospitals, but you will usually be offered a succession of interventions, designed to bring on active labour.

Medical **methods of encouraging the cervix to ripen** include:

- a membrane sweep and/or
- drugs called **prostaglandins** (usually in the form of a pessary or gel) or
- mechanical dilation methods (Foley/double-balloon catheter or laminaria tent)

Medical **methods of strengthening or starting contractions** include:

- **ARM** (breaking the waters) and/or
- synthetic **oxytocin**, given through a drip.

Medical induction processes are carried out in an obstetric unit. The only exception is a membrane sweep (see below) which may be offered at your antenatal appointments wherever those normally take place.

Sometimes the methods used to ripen the cervix are enough by themselves to bring on active labour, but if you are not having strong, regular contractions after these have been tried it's common to be offered **ARM** and/or an **oxytocin** drip. These may also be offered later if your labour is considered by your midwife or doctor to be progressing too slowly.

It's important to be aware that though some people will reach active labour quickly, it is quite common for it to take several days.

A medical induction is more likely to work if you are already close to going into labour. A midwife will usually assess your **Bishop's score** (see below) just before starting a medical induction. You may want to know your score before you decide whether to have a membrane sweep or book a medical induction.

What is the Bishop's score and why is it important?

The **Bishop's score** is an estimate of how close labour is to starting, based on how far the baby has moved down into the pelvis and the progress of the changes in the cervix in preparation for labour to begin. It therefore provides information about how likely a medical induction is to work, and how much progress there has been towards active labour following an induction.

Different hospitals may use slightly different scoring systems, but it is usually reckoned that a score of eight or more means that there is a good chance of a medical induction being effective and leading to a vaginal birth. If the score is very low, it's probably going to take longer for medical methods to work, and there is a higher chance that they won't work at all. Midwives may not think to tell you what your score is, so you may need to ask for this information.

If your score is high it also means that there's a good chance you will go into labour soon anyway, without the need for medical induction. If you have no immediate concerns about the well-being of you or your baby, you could choose to wait a while to see whether your labour begins, and perhaps try non-medical methods of induction during this time (see above).

Midwives may ask to repeat the **Bishop's score** assessment during a medical induction to see whether you are going into labour, but you have the right to decline at any time – even if it is hospital policy for examinations to be performed at set intervals.

As with any medical procedure there are benefits and possible repercussions to having your **Bishop's score** assessed during an induction:

»   It may be helpful for you to know the result to help you decide what to do next.

»   Hearing how far you have progressed could be reassuring.

»   If things haven't moved on very far that could be demoralising.

»   Your midwife will need to perform an internal vaginal examination, and many people find these examinations distressing, uncomfortable or even painful.

You may prefer to rely on other signs of how your labour is progressing. For example:

»   Are you experiencing regular labour contractions, and if so, are they becoming longer, more powerful and closer together over time?

»   Have your waters broken spontaneously?

»   Is your baby moving further down into your pelvis? (You may be aware of this or your midwife can check by feeling your bump.

»   What are your instincts telling you about what is happening in your body?

Membrane sweeping

A membrane sweep may help to stimulate the release of **prostaglandins** and so promote ripening of the cervix in preparation for labour. Though it is a method of induction it is often treated as a routine procedure for anyone who has not gone into labour by a certain number of weeks of pregnancy.

The NICE guideline on Inducing Labour (NICE 2008) currently recommend that first-time mothers should be offered a sweep at their antenatal appointments at 40 and 41 weeks, and those who have birthed before should be offered one at 41 weeks, but some places will offer it earlier than this. A sweep may also be offered in hospital as the first step in a medical induction.

Your midwife or doctor may assume that you will agree to a sweep, but as with any procedure, they should provide you with clear information about the benefits and risks and accept your decision if you decline.

To perform a sweep, a midwife or doctor carries out an internal vaginal examination, and at the same time passes a finger inside the cervix and moves it around to loosen the membranes that surround the amniotic fluid in which the baby floats.

However, if the cervix has yet to move forwards it may be difficult for the midwife or doctor to reach it. Sometimes changing your position would be enough to bring your cervix far enough forward for a sweep but if it remains far back (posterior) an attempt to do a sweep may be very uncomfortable and may not be possible. If it can be reached but is tightly closed the midwife will not be able to do a sweep but may offer to massage around it. It's not known whether this has any effect, and it should be noted that a tightly closed cervix may well be a sign that your body is not yet ready to labour.

Remember that you can ask your midwife about your **Bishop's score** before deciding whether to go ahead with a sweep.

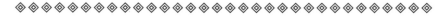

Research Evidence

A review of the research evidence (Boulvain 2005) concluded that having a sweep at term (after 40 weeks) reduces the number of pregnancies that last beyond 42 weeks but that for one mother to avoid medical induction on the grounds of length of pregnancy seven others would have had sweeps that had no such effect.

The review also found that having a sweep may result in labour and birth occurring about three days sooner on average than they would otherwise have done, although some of the larger studies included in the review did not find such a clear effect.

In one study, for example, membrane sweeping from 39 weeks of pregnancy if the **Bishop's score** was low did *not* increase the chances of going into labour before 41 weeks. (Putnam, 2011). This suggests that a sweep may only be effective if you are close to going into labour anyway.

The Boulvain review concluded "For women near term (37 to 40 weeks of gestation) in an uncomplicated pregnancy there seems to be little justification for performing routine sweeping of membranes."

The review also found that women who had sweeps reported that they were more painful than other vaginal examinations, and sweeps seemed to be more likely to result in vaginal bleeding and painful contractions that do not lead to active labour.

» » »» » »»» » »» » »» » »» » »» » »» » »» » »» » »» » » » »» » » »

Summary

> » A membrane sweep may bring on labour sooner than it would otherwise have started. However, the evidence indicates that it may only be effective if you are close to going into labour anyway.

> » It requires a vaginal examination, which you may find painful or distressing. It may also cause vaginal bleeding and ineffective painful contractions.

> » If you are content to wait for labour to start naturally, when your baby is ready, you may want to decline a routine sweep, but if you are being advised to have your labour induced and you have reason to want your baby to be born soon you may consider a sweep helpful.

Things to consider

- Do you have a reason for wanting to try to get your labour started a bit sooner, or are you happy to wait for it to happen in its own time?

- Would you like to be told your **Bishop's score** before deciding whether to have a sweep (bearing in mind that this would mean having two vaginal examinations if you decide to go ahead with the sweep)?

- Are you aware of any signs which suggest that your labour will start soon? (*See "Signs that your body is preparing for labour", p.106.*)

Induction with Prostaglandin

The **prostaglandin** which is used in a medical induction is chemically the same as the one that is naturally produced to start the process of ripening the cervix, but it is applied artificially. It is administered in hospital, though depending on the circumstances you can choose to go home after being given it.

Normally, before giving you prostaglandin your midwife will want to assess your **Bishop's score** and may offer to do a membrane sweep at the same time. Midwives tend to assume that if you have agreed to a medical induction you will automatically accept vaginal examinations at intervals through the process, but you have the right to decline any or all of them.

After this, the midwife will insert a preparation of the prostaglandin into your vagina. There are different types including pessaries (in the form of a tablet or gel) which last for about 6-8 hours, or a slow-release version which carries on releasing the drug for up to 24 hours. You may want to find out in advance which your hospital normally uses.

You can be offered a second or sometimes a third dose of the shorter-lasting preparations if you haven't started to have strong regular labour contractions within 6-8 hours of the previous dose. Before a repeat dose, your midwife will probably want to do another vaginal examination to see whether there are signs that your cervix is ripening, or if it has started to dilate. It is up to you whether you feel that an additional examination would give you useful information about the progress of your labour, or if you would prefer to decline it.

In a slow-release pessary the drug is contained in a thin plastic casing with a tape to remove it. This can be left in for up to 24 hours or removed earlier if you have started to have strong, regular contractions. If your labour hasn't started after 24 hours with the slow-release pessary in place, you may be offered one or more doses of one of the other preparations.

Prostaglandin can bring on sudden, strong contractions which can be stressful for the baby, so it's normal to suggest **continuous monitoring** of your baby's heartbeat for a short period (typically 20-30 minutes) after the first dose is given. If the process causes your baby to become distressed the induction will need to be stopped, and you may need to consider having a **caesarean**.

However, if all is well after the initial monitoring period your midwife should just offer to listen to your baby's heartbeat from time to time with a stethoscope or hand-held monitor. That means that there is no need for you to stay in the antenatal ward the whole time. You might choose to go out for a stroll, or to sit in the hospital cafe. Increasingly, women who are using the slow-release pessary are choosing to go home and relax for 24 hours or until labour starts, if there are no complicating factors. This is sometimes referred to as out-patient induction.

If you are planning a VBAC (vaginal birth after caesarean) there are other possible risks to consider – *see "VBAC labour", p.96.*

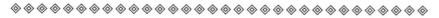

Research Evidence

There is some evidence from a recent review (Thomas *et al*, 2014) that having prostaglandin may increase the chances of giving birth vaginally within 24 hours. The main trial on which the authors based this conclusion (Egarter 1989) only included women with a **Bishop's score** of over 4. Another trial (Ulmsten 1985), which only included women with a very low Bishop's score, found that prostaglandin made no difference. This means we can't be sure if prostaglandin will be effective in inducing labour in a short time, if at all, if the Bishop's score is low. Many people have found that it took considerably longer than 24 hours after the first dose of prostaglandin before labour even began. This may have been because they had a low **Bishop's score** at the start of the induction.

In some cases, giving prostaglandin over-stimulates the womb muscles (called uterine hyperstimulation). This is defined as either very long contractions (lasting two minutes or more) or very frequent contractions (more than five in 10 minutes). As well as being potentially painful, these very long or very frequent contractions can reduce the amount of blood flowing to the baby, and so may cause the baby to become distressed. The Thomas 2014 review discussed above estimated that this might affect around one in 20 women who have induction with prostaglandin. Most cases of hyperstimulation can be treated effectively without lasting harm to the baby, but in about two in every 100 cases of hyperstimulation the baby needs to be born by **caesarean** (Egarter 1990). That means that about one in 1,000 babies of mothers who receive prostaglandin will need to be born swiftly by caesarean.

Some people experience nausea and sharp pains (sometimes called 'Prostin pains' after a trade-name for prostaglandin).

» » »» » »» » »» » »» » »» » »» » »» » »» » »» » »» » » » »» » » »

Summary

» Giving prostaglandin may be effective in bringing on labour, and for some people it seems to increase the chance of giving birth within 24 hours, but for others it may take much longer. We can't be sure, but this seems likely to be related to whether their **Bishop's score** was high or low.

» The drug can cause severe pain and nausea, and about 5% of people who have it will experience very long or very frequent contractions.

» This hyperstimulation of the womb muscles can cause babies to become distressed and it is normal to have **continuous monitoring** of your baby's heartbeat for 20 or 30 minutes after insertion of prostaglandin.

» One in 1,000 babies may not respond to treatment for this and you may need an unplanned **caesarean** as a result.

Mechanical dilation methods

Mechanical methods to open the cervix were used before the development of prostaglandin pessaries and now seem to be coming back into favour, although their use is still relatively uncommon. The NICE guideline on Inducing Labour (NICE 2008) says that they should not be used routinely, but a more recent Interventional Procedures Guideline (NICE 2015) says that there is now evidence to support the use of a double-balloon (Foley) catheter.

In this method a catheter (a thin plastic tube) with one or two balloons around it is placed inside the cervix then the balloons are slowly filled with saline solution (water with salt dissolved in it) to gently push the cervix open. Another, less common, method is a laminaria tent. This is made up of several rods of dried seaweed which are inserted into the cervix. They gradually absorb moisture, causing them to expand. In both cases the pressure is thought to stimulate the release of the natural prostaglandin as well as mechanically dilating the cervix.

Use of double-balloon catheter for induction

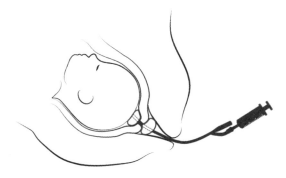

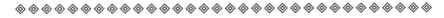

Research Evidence

There is some evidence that using mechanical methods can be as effective as using prostaglandin, and that there is less risk of them overstimulating the muscles of the womb (Jozwiak 2012). You might want to discuss using one of these mechanical methods of induction instead of prostaglandin.

Most of the studies that have been done were small, and not all reported on the effectiveness of the method. Those which compared balloon catheters with prostaglandin found no difference between the methods in the number of women who gave birth within 24 hours or who had caesareans – in other words, the methods were equally effective. However, only 11 out of 1000 women who had the catheter method had hyperstimulation which affected the baby's heart rate compared to 31 out of 1000 who had prostaglandin.

For laminaria tents, there seem to be no good quality studies that have looked at their effectiveness compared with prostaglandins, but some that showed **a lower risk of hyperstimulation affecting the baby's heart rate**.

Summary

> » Mechanical methods offer an alternative to prostaglandin for induction. There is some limited evidence that they are equally effective and have less risk of over-stimulating the womb muscles.

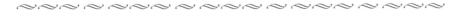

Things to consider

- You should have the choice of what method of medical induction you want to use, so think about what you would prefer.
- How would you feel about having a membrane sweep as the first step in the induction process?
- How do you feel about using prostaglandin compared with using a mechanical method? Which would you prefer?
- If using a mechanical method, would you prefer a Foley (double-balloon) catheter or a laminaria tent? It's worth checking to make sure that your hospital will have your preferred device available for you.

- If using prostaglandin would you prefer to start with a slow-release pessary? If so, you may want to make sure that your hospital will have this available.
- If you are going to have a slow-release prostaglandin pessary, would you want to go home after this has been inserted if all is well or would you prefer to stay in hospital?

Breaking the waters (amniotomy/ARM)

Sometimes the use of **prostaglandin** or a mechanical method is enough to bring on effective labour contractions and nothing further is needed. If not, once the cervix is slightly dilated, midwives and doctors will often suggest breaking the waters to try to start or strengthen the contractions. This is sometimes referred to as an amniotomy or artificial rupture of the membranes (**ARM**).

It is a common experience that contractions become a lot stronger after the waters break naturally during labour. This may be because it allows the baby's head to move down and press on the lower part of the womb, which sends signals to the brain telling it to produce more **oxytocin**. **ARM** is intended to mimic this process but there is no direct evidence to show whether **ARM** following a medical induction is helpful or does more harm than good.

ARM is done using a sterile plastic device like a large crochet hook (an amnihook) which is inserted into the vagina and through the cervix to nick the membranes around the amniotic fluid.

Midwives and doctors are often keen to move on to this intervention once the cervix has dilated enough for them to do it, and hospital guidelines may encourage this. However, as with any other medical intervention, it is your decision whether to agree to ARM or to consider alternatives. These might include waiting longer, having (another) dose of prostaglandin, or having a caesarean.

It's usual to be admitted to a birth room before ARM is done. This can mean that, if the induction is not considered urgent and all the rooms are busy, you may have to wait for quite some time – hours or occasionally days – until a birth room is free.

Like a vaginal examination, ARM can be uncomfortable or painful. Those who have ARM sometimes report that it resulted in a sudden and unmanageable increase in the strength of their contractions. If this happens it could put more stress on your baby and affect their heart rate. Because of this you will usually be recommended to have **continuous monitoring** after ARM which may restrict your mobility. As with all interventions you can decline this.

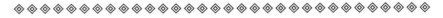

Research Evidence

There is very little evidence about the safety and effectiveness of using ARM to speed up the process of induction. The NICE guidelines (NICE 2008) say "Amniotomy (ARM), alone or with oxytocin, should not be used as a primary method of induction of labour unless there are specific clinical reasons for not using vaginal PGE2" (i.e. prostaglandin). In other words, it isn't recommended as a way of starting labour, but they say nothing about using it if you are not in active labour after using prostaglandin or a mechanical method.

A recent Cochrane review of evidence for breaking the waters to speed up a spontaneous labour (Smyth 2013) does not support doing this, either routinely in normally progressing spontaneous labour or where labours have become prolonged. Routine use of ARM did not appear to shorten the time it took for the cervix to dilate fully or to reduce the number of mothers who had an unplanned **caesarean**. It also was not shown to improve the health of babies in these situations.

The review did not look at the effects of breaking the waters to try to bring on active labour following induction, so we can't tell whether it is helpful in that situation or not.

Though the authors of the review comment that "There are a number of potential important but rare risks associated with amniotomy, including problems with the umbilical cord or the baby's heart rate" they did not find a **statistically significant** difference in any of these whether or not amniotomy was used in a spontaneous labour.

» » »» » »» » »» » »» » »» » »» » »» » »» » »» » »» » » » »» » » »

Summary

  » Despite its widespread use there is no direct evidence that **ARM** helps progress into active labour following induction. As the review (Smyth 2013) mentioned above does not recommend its routine use in spontaneous labours it is reasonable to question why this should be any different for a labour which has been started artificially.

  » There are some potential risks which include pain, increased stress on mother and baby, infection and possibly the rare risk of cord prolapse.

  » Having **ARM** will mean **continuous monitoring** will be recommended.

Synthetic oxytocin (Syntocinon, Pitocin)

If active labour has not begun within a short time after breaking the waters (ARM), most hospitals will offer to give you synthetic **oxytocin** through a drip to try to speed things up. How soon it is offered will depend on hospital policy, and some places offer it at the same time as ARM. In any case it is up to you whether you want to have this immediately, wait a bit longer and try other ways to encourage your labour to progress, or request a **caesarean**.

Synthetic oxytocin (known in the UK by the trade name Syntocinon and in the USA as Pitocin) is given through a needle in your hand or arm attached via a tube to a pump on a drip stand. It is an artificially manufactured version of the hormone which is produced in spontaneous labour to start and maintain labour contractions. The amount of the drug being given will be increased until you are having strong and frequent contractions.

Synthetic oxytocin is a powerful drug and it is often given in doses much higher than the manufacturer recommends. As this could have consequences for you and your baby, you may want to make it clear that you only consent to it being used within the licensed dosage range. For more on this see *www.aims.org.uk/journal/item/unlicensed-oxytocin-doses*.

The sudden increase in strength of contractions caused by synthetic oxytocin can be stressful for both mother and baby. It increases the chance that signs of distress will be seen in the baby's heartbeat (Bugg 2013), though most babies will cope with it without problems. Turning down or stopping the drip will usually relieve the problem quickly. This is why it is recommended that the baby's heartbeat is monitored continuously once the drip has been put up. If a baby becomes seriously distressed, they may need to be born by **caesarean** or with the assistance of **forceps** or **ventouse**.

Stronger contractions can also be hard to cope with, so you should be offered an **epidural** at the same time, though not everyone finds that they need this (Alfirevic 2009). Make sure that your midwife discusses this with you and arranges it if you want it. An epidural can itself increase the chances of instruments being used to assist the birth (Anim-Somuah M, 2018). (More information about epidurals is on the AIMS Birth Information web page *www.aims.org.uk/information/item/managing-labour.)*

Women often report that a labour induced or **augmented** with synthetic oxytocin feels very different from one which is progressing spontaneously. Although synthetic oxytocin has the same effect on the womb muscles as the natural hormone, it does not seem to have the same effect on the mother's mood and ability to manage her labour. It has been suggested that this is because natural oxytocin is produced in the brain in high concentrations and so has a strong 'feel-good' effect there (Buckley 2011). In contrast, when the artificial variety is given directly into the bloodstream this switches off the natural production and little if any crosses back from the mother's bloodstream to her brain (Bell 2014).

If you know you have a heart condition the use of synthetic oxytocin should be discussed with your heart specialist as well as your obstetrician, so you can decide whether this would be safe for you if it was to be offered.

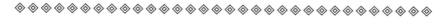

Research Evidence

Most of the trials that have been done have compared using synthetic oxytocin with using prostaglandin to start the process of induction. It seems to be less effective than prostaglandin and to have more side effects including more caesareans, more heavy bleeding after birth and lower satisfaction for mothers (Howarth & Botha 2001, Alfirevic 2009, Mozurkewich 2011). This is why NICE does not recommend it as a first step in a medical induction.

No one seems to have investigated the effect of synthetic oxytocin on the progress of a labour after prostaglandin or a mechanical method have been used, despite the frequency with which this is offered.

For labours that have started spontaneously, but are progressing slowly, there is some evidence that an oxytocin drip can reduce the length of labour by an average of about two hours (Bugg 2013). As mentioned earlier (*p.105*), for first-time mothers the active stage of labour (when the cervix is dilating from 4cm to 10cm) lasts on average eight hours and is unlikely to last over 18 hours. For those who have birthed before, the same stage will last on average five hours and is unlikely to last over 12 hours. An oxytocin drip doesn't seem to reduce the chances of a **caesarean** or **assisted birth** in a spontaneous labour.

For labours that have been induced, we don't know whether an oxytocin drip would reduce the length or affect the chances of a caesarean or assisted birth because the research has not been done.

Studies which compared immediate use of an oxytocin drip with waiting for eight hours when progress in labour was considered too slow, found that in just under seven in 100 mothers in the oxytocin group the baby had signs of distress which required action, compared with fewer than three mothers in the other group. (Bugg 2013)

It is possible that synthetic oxytocin use can have other effects on the well-being of mothers and babies, though the evidence about this is limited. One analysis (Buchanan 2012) looked at how many mothers and babies suffered health problems after birth according to whether they were exposed synthetic oxytocin during labour. The researchers used so-called 'composite indicators' of poor health, which combine a range of diseases (like breathing problems, heart problems or infections) and treatments (such as ventilation, blood transfusion or surgery) that mothers or babies may experience after birth.

For all mothers in the study, if synthetic oxytocin was not given around 3% of babies and 1.3% of mothers suffered one or more of these problems; with synthetic oxytocin babies this rose to about 4% of babies and 2% of mothers. Where induction or **augmentation** was not being done because of an existing concern over the mother's or baby's health, the picture was very similar. The authors therefore concluded that synthetic oxytocin causes an increase in health problems, that isn't due simply to pre-existing medical problems.

A recent **population study** in Massachusetts (Kroll-Desrosiers 2017) found that mothers who had had synthetic oxytocin during labour had a higher chance of developing **postnatal depression** in the first year than those who did not, regardless of the type of birth they had.

» » »» » »» » »» » »» » »» » »» » »» » »» » »» » »» » » » »» » » »

Summary

» There is some evidence that an oxytocin drip is effective in shortening labour by around two hours on average. It doesn't seem to reduce the need for a **caesarean** or **assisted birth**. The evidence we have concerns spontaneous labours, so we can't be sure that the effects will be the same in a labour started by medical induction.

» Synthetic oxytocin may make labour more difficult and stressful.

» If you choose to have an **epidural** for pain relief, this in turn may increase the likelihood of needing help with forceps or ventouse to give birth.

» An oxytocin drip also increases the chance that your baby will show signs of distress, and therefore you will be recommended to have **continuous monitoring**.

» There may be other short or long term consequences for mother's and baby's well-being, but as yet we don't have enough evidence to be sure about this.

What are my options during an induction?

People sometimes talk as if once the process of induction has begun, a whole series of interventions is inevitable (the so-called 'cascade of interventions'). Although this is a common experience, others find that the first one or two steps in the process are effective, and they then labour without further interventions and have straightforward vaginal births.

If you don't go into labour quickly there are options at each stage which you may want to consider. These could include waiting a bit longer before moving on to the next step, trying self-help methods or complementary therapies *(see "Non-medical forms of induction", p.106)* or in some cases repeating the step (for example, having a further dose of prostaglandin).

As the chart below shows, there are points during an induction at which different courses of action are possible or could be tried in succession. These include:

- If after several prostaglandin treatments your cervix has not started to dilate.
- If your cervix has started to dilate but you are not yet in active labour.
- If your waters have been broken but you still aren't in active labour.

Some people will decide to have their baby by **caesarean** as an alternative to medical induction, or if their labour has still not started after one or more steps. A caesarean might also be recommended at any stage before or during an induction if there was a cause for serious concern about the baby's well-being or ability to cope with further interventions.

You can find out more about the comparative risks of vaginal and caesarean birth in the NICE caesarean guidelines (NICE 2011) *www.nice.org. uk/guidance/cg132/ifp/chapter/Risks-of-caesarean-section* and in this article on the AIMS website *www.aims.org.uk/information/item/caesarean*.

Induction Decision Points

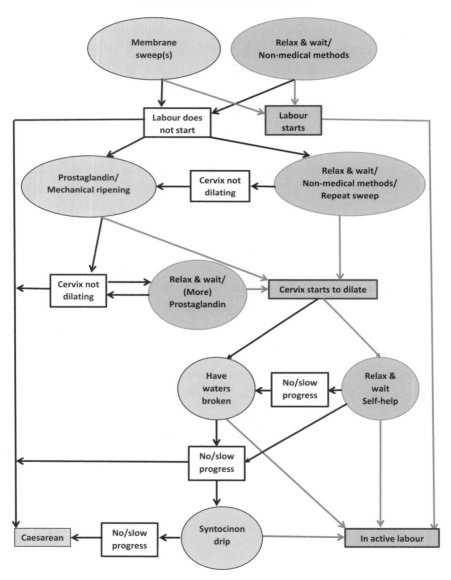

Deciding on the right course of action for you at each stage will depend on things like:

- Are you and your baby currently OK?
- What is your **Bishop's score** now and how has it changed since the induction process started?
- Are there other signs that your labour has started or about how it is progressing? What are your instincts telling you about this?
- If you decided to wait a while before going on to the next step, would that increase the risks for you or your baby, and if so by how much?
- How well has your baby coped with the induction so far, and are there any reasons to think they might start to cope less well as time goes on?
- How well have you coped with the induction so far, how tired are you and how do you feel about continuing? Might it help to take a rest for a while before you decide?
- What are your preferences about having further interventions or having a **caesarean** at this point?

If you are already in strong labour, or under the influence of pain-killing drugs, or just very tired, it can be hard to consider these questions. In addition, having to think and talk, and the stress of worrying about making the right decision, may reduce your production of natural **oxytocin**. This could prevent labour from starting or slow it down if it has begun. It may therefore be helpful to think through in advance what your preferences would be in different situations.

If you expect to have care in labour from a named midwife (or one of a small team) who you are seeing for you antenatal care then you can talk your preferences over with them and agree a **birth plan**. Otherwise, you might want a written birth plan to share with the midwives you see during your labour. It can also be useful if your partner or other birth supporter can discuss any need for a decision which arises during labour with your midwife or doctor and then summarise it for you, rather than you having to engage in complicated discussions.

Most midwives and doctors tend to assume that if active labour has not begun after one intervention, you will automatically go on to the next one. However, even if you have agreed to induction, they should check whether you give informed consent to any other procedures which you may be offered later. The Royal College of Obstetricians and Gynaecologists' guidelines on "Obtaining Valid Consent" (RCOG 2015b) says, "If a procedure is planned {during labour} she should receive a full explanation as if she had not previously had the relevant information... Women should be encouraged to express their views on such procedures so that their carers are aware of the choices made by the women and act accordingly." It may also be helpful to remember that even if you have given your consent at the start of the induction process you have the right to withdraw it at any time *(see "Informed consent" on p.1)*.

If want to do something different from your hospital's standard practice then you may have to be assertive about asking to review all the options. A helpful question can be "Is this an emergency, or have we got time to talk about what to do next?" This can remind your midwife or doctor that they should be enabling you to make an informed decision, without assuming what that decision will be. If you are writing a birth plan it may be helpful to include a statement that you would like to discuss things at each stage before deciding whether to move on to further interventions.

As with all decisions, it can be useful to apply 'BRAIN' *(see p.7* or AIMS Birth Information web page, *www.aims.org.uk/information/item/making-decisions)*, ask questions to get all the information that you need, and if you feel it would be helpful, ask for a second opinion.

What may help an induction to work?

Labour, whether spontaneous or medically induced, is more likely to start and then to progress to active labour in circumstances that encourage your body to produce the right mix of labour hormones: **oxytocin** to stimulate contractions and encourage a feeling of well-being, and endorphins, the body's 'natural painkillers' which also help to reduce stress and bring feelings of pleasure (Buckley 2011).

You are more likely to produce these helpful hormones when you feel safe, supported and relaxed. Anything that makes you anxious, or disturbs your privacy is likely to increase your adrenaline levels which in turn will reduce your production of oxytocin and thus slow down or completely stop contractions, especially in the first stage (Buckley 2011). This can happen if people are talking alarmingly about risks to your baby's well-being, or because you are in a strange place, surrounded by people you do not know while being constantly monitored and checked.

What all this means is that your labour is likely to be shorter, and induction methods are more likely to be effective, if you are well-supported and (as far as possible) can put any worries out of your mind.

There is also good evidence that having continuous support during labour can increase your chances of a straightforward vaginal birth, make your labour slightly shorter, reduce your need for drugs for pain relief and make it more likely that your baby is in good condition at birth (Bohren 2017).

Birth supporters can help by making sure that you are disturbed as little as possible and by giving you reassurance and encouragement, as well as reminding you to take care of your own well-being, for example resting when tired, eating and drinking to keep up your energy, and finding comfortable positions. Walking around and using upright positions has been shown to reduce the length of labour, the chances of a caesarean, and the need for **epidural** pain relief (Lawrence 2013).

You may like to experiment and find some ways of relaxing which will help to calm your mind and encourage your labour hormones to flow. Different methods will work for different people, but you may find things like yoga, hypnobirthing, breathing techniques and massage helpful. Bright lights tend to disturb labour, so dimming the lights, or using an eye mask if that isn't possible, may help.

Helpful things

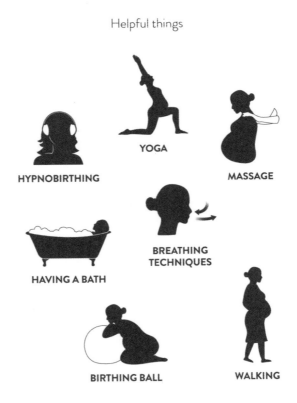

HYPNOBIRTHING

YOGA

MASSAGE

HAVING A BATH

BREATHING
TECHNIQUES

BIRTHING BALL

WALKING

» » »» » »» » »» » »» » »» » »» » »» » »» » »» » » » »» » » »

Summary

- » There are many ways which you can use to encourage the progress of your labour, and these are likely to be helpful when labour is being induced as well as when it starts spontaneously.
- » Anything which helps you to relax and to feel safe should encourage your labour hormones to flow.
- » There is good evidence that continuous support, walking around and using upright positions increase your chances of having a straightforward birth.

How does an induction differ from a spontaneous labour?

Having an induced labour can be very different from being in spontaneous labour. You won't necessarily experience all the possibilities listed below but being prepared for them may help you to feel more in control and increase your chances of an otherwise straightforward birth. You may also find it helpful to think about them in advance or write a **birth plan** about how you would like to manage these situations if they occur.

An induction limits your options for where to give birth

Medical inductions (apart from membrane sweeps) are only carried out in a hospital obstetric unit, so agreeing to induction means that going to a birth centre is no longer an option.

If all is well after the insertion of a prostaglandin pessary or mechanical induction device you may prefer to go home. In fact, hospitals are increasingly recommending this, especially when a slow-release prostaglandin pessary is used. However, you will be advised to return to hospital for monitoring either after a certain number of hours or once labour begins, whichever is sooner.

Legally, you still have the right to have a homebirth in this situation, but midwives are likely to be reluctant to support this after starting an induction. **ARM** or starting an **oxytocin** drip will only be done in hospital.

Induction may take days

Many people do not realise that it is very unlikely that their baby will be born on the date that the induction process is started, and in fact it could be as much as four or five days later.

It's common to have two or three doses of prostaglandin at six- or eight-hourly intervals, or the slow-release pessary for 24 hours possibly followed by one or more doses of gel. During this time, you may feel as though nothing is happening, though in fact the ripening of your cervix may be progressing. Alternatively, you may start experiencing mild labour contractions, or the more severe 'Prostin pains' during this time.

There can be a delay before your waters are broken or an oxytocin drip started as these procedures are normally only done in the birth room. If the hospital is busy, other people who have arrived in strong labour will be admitted to birth rooms ahead of you.

All of this can mean that you may already be tired and stressed by the time active labour begins, especially if you were not expecting things to take so long. It's worth making sure that you rest when you are tired, and eat and drink as you want to, so that you will have the energy to labour effectively once things get going. It can be a good idea to pack plenty of drinks and snacks for you and your supporter(s).

If the induction is taking a long time, it may be helpful to use the time to relax and prepare to greet your baby. This may be easier if you have gone home after the start of the induction process, but even if there is a reason for staying at the hospital you could sit outside, go for a walk, or go to a nearby coffee shop rather than to stay on the antenatal ward all the time. You might like to take something to occupy your mind (knitting, reading, games, films to watch…) and some personal pictures or objects that have positive associations for you. You could also practice in advance some self-help methods you and your supporter(s) might use to help you stay calm, like relaxed breathing, massage or hypnobirthing techniques.

Support on the antenatal ward may be limited

During the time that you are on the antenatal ward, depending on the hospital's practices, the support that is available to you may be limited.

It is common to be attended on the antenatal ward by a midwife who is caring for several women so you may only see her at intervals of several hours. If you need anything, you should have a call button to ask for attention.

Ideally everyone having their labours induced should be accompanied throughout by one or more birth supporters of their choice, but often hospital staff do not want partners or other supporters to stay in the antenatal ward overnight or may suggest that they go home and rest until active labour begins. This can mean being left with little or no support at a time when you might really need it. You may want to see whether you can arrange for someone to be with you, at least during the daytime and preferably throughout the induction process and your labour. This factsheet from the charity Birthrights, *www.birthrights.org.uk/library/factsheets/Birth-Partners.pdf,* sets out your legal rights on choosing birth supporters, and says, "Whenever a hospital policy is applied to you, health practitioners must take account of your personal needs and consider making exceptions to the policy if they are required" – especially if you have additional physical or cultural needs. Some people refuse to agree to an induction unless their personal needs for support are met.

Pain relief options

Having an induction may limit the types of pain relief that are available especially in the early stages.

You will be able to use self-help methods including a TENS machine, massage, a bath or shower, or complementary therapies like hypnotherapy, aromatherapy, acupuncture/acupressure or homeopathy while on the antenatal ward, but probably won't have access to Entonox (gas and air) or an **epidural**. Some hospitals have midwives trained in alternative therapies, but you may need to do some practice or buy some materials beforehand if you plan to use any of these, and you may need a supporter to help you.

An option that is more likely to be available on an antenatal ward is an injection of an opiate drug like Pethidine. People react to this in different ways. Some will find it helps them to relax and even sleep, but not everyone finds it effective or likes the way it makes them feel.

Once you have been admitted to a birth room, you should have more options for managing your labour, including Entonox, a birthpool or an epidural (but see below for use of birth pools if having **continuous monitoring** or on a drip).

For more on ways of managing labour see the AIMS Birth Information article on *www.aims.org.uk/information/item/managing-labour*.

Continuous monitoring is likely to be recommended

Due to the possible side effects of prostaglandin, it's usually suggested that the baby's heartbeat is continuously monitored with a cardiotocography machine (CTG) for a short period after the drug is inserted. The monitors are then removed if all is well.

If you have your waters broken or an oxytocin drip you will usually be advised to have continuous monitoring for the rest of your labour to check for any problems. (See the AIMS Birth Information web page "Monitoring your baby's heartbeat in labour", *www.aims.org.uk/information/item/monitoring-your-babys-heartbeat-in-labour.*

Being connected to a monitor may limit your ability to move around and change position, but it should be possible for you to be monitored in a range of upright positions. Despite what you may have seen on the television (and what some midwives or doctors will say) there is no need to sit or lie on a bed just because you are being monitored or have a drip inserted.

It is possible to use a birthpool even with continuous monitoring if the hospital has telemetry equipment that lets the midwife monitor the baby's heartbeat remotely, but some hospitals are reluctant to allow this.

Induction is likely to involve multiple vaginal examinations
Hospital induction guidelines usually require the midwife to carry out repeated vaginal examinations to check what progress there has been. You have a right to decide whether to accept every one that is offered, but may find that a midwife will not admit you to a birth room or carry out the next step of the induction unless you agree to one.

Another issue is that often a midwife will ask you to lie down while she examines you. If your contractions have started by then, this can make them harder to manage, so a you might want to ask your midwife to examine you in a position which you find comfortable. For more about vaginal examinations see the AIMS Birth Information web page "Vaginal examinations in Labour", *www.aims.org.uk/information/item/vaginal-examinations-in-labour.*

Planning for an induction of labour

If you know that your labour is likely to be induced, you can think in advance about the decisions you might need to make and what you, your midwives and your birth supporters can do to help. It may be helpful to discuss some of these with your own midwife beforehand and/or make a note of them to share with the midwives who will be caring for you.

If you are writing a **birth plan** say that if your labour is being induced, you would like to discuss things at each stage before deciding whether to move on to further interventions.

Questions you might want to ask beforehand

Hospitals' standard procedures for induction and the options available vary quite a lot, so find out as much as you can from your hospital:

- What time of day do they suggest that you come in to have an induction of labour started? Evidence suggests that it doesn't make much difference to the outcome, but mothers tend to prefer the morning (NICE 2008).

- Which methods do they use for cervical ripening – a slow release **prostaglandin** pessary, a standard prostaglandin pessary or mechanical methods (Foley catheter and/or laminaria tent)?

- What are their protocols for induction? They should have an information leaflet which explains this, or you could ask for copies of their guidelines. Things you might want to know include:

  » Do they do an initial membrane sweep on admission? If so, how soon after that would they expect to insert prostaglandin or start a mechanical method?

  » Do they start with a slow release prostaglandin pessary?

  » How many doses of prostaglandin would they give before considering other courses of action?

> » Do they normally start an **oxytocin** drip at the same time as **ARM**, or wait a few hours to see whether active labour begins without the drip?
> » When would they suggest starting **continuous monitoring**?

- Would they encourage you to go home in the early stages of induction, if there is no agreed need for continuous monitoring?
- What facilities are there for you in the early stages of induction? Is there somewhere to walk around outside? Is there a café, restaurant, or kitchen that you can use?
- What are their guidelines on partners or other supporters being with you while having induction on the antenatal ward?
- What methods of pain relief are available to you on the antenatal ward?
- What are their guidelines on the use of a birth pool (if available) for an induced labour?
- If you are having an **oxytocin** drip, an **epidural** and/or continuous monitoring will you be encouraged/enabled to be mobile and use helpful positions for labour?

Things you may want to discuss

- If you are not happy with the time of day (morning or evening) that your hospital plans to start your induction you can ask whether it could be started at a different time.
- If you have a preference for the method to be used to ripen your cervix ask for it to be made available.
- Do you want to take some time to consider your options rather than automatically proceeding to the next step of your hospital's standard induction process? *(See "What are my options during an induction?" p.123.)* If so, you may need to make sure that your midwives and doctors are aware of this, and that you or your supporters remind them as appropriate.

- Do you want to have your **Bishop's score** and its implications explained to you before deciding on the next step?
- If your hospital normally restricts the times that partners or other supporters can be on the antenatal ward, do you want to negotiate to have someone with you? It may be possible to argue for this if you have a specific need, for example if you have a disability, suffer from severe anxiety or if English is not your first language.
- If your hospital does not normally make a birth pool available when the labour has been induced, you could negotiate to use one. Again, some people will decline induction if this would prevent them from using a birthpool.

Things you may want to think about

- Would you want to go home in the early stages of induction if all is well with you and your baby, or would you prefer to be in hospital?
- If it takes several days before you are in active labour, how can you make sure you get enough to eat and drink during this time? You may need to check whether they can provide for any specific dietary requirements that you have. You might want to see if there is a café/restaurant or a kitchen you can use, or you might decide to pack your own food or arrange for someone bring it in for you.
- What might help you to rest and sleep e.g. eye masks, headphones, hypnobirthing recordings, having your own pillow?
- What methods might you want to use or what can your supporters to do to help you cope with early labour while you are on the antenatal ward? *(See "What may help an induction to work?" p.127.)*
- If initial attempts to induce your labour are not successful would you be happy to keep going with further interventions, or would you want to stop and wait for a while (assuming you and your baby are well)?
- If attempts to induce your labour are not successful would you be happy to keep going with further interventions, or is there a point at which you would prefer to switch to a **caesarean** (e.g. rather

than having **ARM** or an **oxytocin** drip?)

- If you are having an oxytocin drip do you want to have an **epidural** put in at the same time, or wait and see how you get on without it?
- How can you prepare yourself mentally for the possibility that induction may take several days to work?
- How can you prepare yourself for the possibility that the induction may fail, and your baby need to be born by caesarean?

Resources

For useful links, research updates and other resources see the web page
www.aims.org.uk/general/induction

Glossary

Absolute Risk is the chance of a problem occurring, usually expressed as one in 100, one in 1000 etc.

ARM (artificial rupture of the membranes) is a method of **augmentation** in which a midwife or doctor breaks the membranes which surround the baby in the womb using a special device. This requires an internal vaginal examination.

Assisted birth is a birth which is assisted by a doctor using either **forceps** or a **ventouse** to help get a baby out of the birth canal by turning and/or pulling on the baby's head while the mother pushes. This may be offered if:

- The second ('pushing') stage of labour has gone on for a long time.
- A baby's head is not in a good position for birth and needs to be turned
- If there are signs that a baby is not coping well during this stage.

For more information on this including the pros and cons of forceps and ventouse see *www.nhs.uk/conditions/pregnancy-and-baby/ventouse-forceps-delivery/*

Augmentation is the use of medical procedures (**ARM** and/or a synthetic **oxytocin** drip) intended to start or strengthen labour contractions. These may be used as part of the process of induction following the use of prostaglandin or a mechanical method. They may also be used to try to speed up a labour which started spontaneously, if progress is thought to be too slow.

Birth plan is a statement of your preferences for labour and birth, to share with your midwife.

Bishop's score is an estimate of how close active labour is to starting, based on a midwife's judgement of the following factors:

- Dilation: How far the cervix has opened.
- Effacement: How much the cervix has thinned.
- Station: How far down in the pelvis the baby has moved.
- Consistency: How soft the cervix has become.
- Position: How far forward the cervix is.

The midwife assesses the cervix while performing an internal vaginal examination and feels the bump to work out where baby's head is in relation to the pelvis. The midwife allocates zero, one or two points for how far each of the changes has progressed, then add them up to give a total score. A lot depends on the midwife's judgement, so it's far from an exact science.

Caesarean is a procedure to birth a baby through a surgical opening in the abdomen and womb. You can find out more about the benefits and risks of caesareans in the NICE guidelines (NICE 2011) *www.nice.org.uk/guidance/cg132/ifp/ chapter/Risks-of-caesarean-section* and in this article on the AIMS website *www.aims.org. uk/information/item/caesarean*

Cerebral palsy is the name given to a group of conditions that have a life-long effect on movement and co-ordination. Most cases occur as a result of problems with the development of a baby's brain during pregnancy. It can also be caused by something that damages the brain during labour or soon after birth, such as low oxygen, low blood sugar or an infection like meningitis.

Continuous monitoring is the use of a machine to track how a baby's heart is responding over time and to look back at the history of how the response has changed through labour.

It is usual for a midwife to monitor a baby's heart rate during labour to check how they are responding to labour contractions. For straightforward pregnancies it is recommended that this is done intermittently (from time to time) using either a small stethoscope or a hand-held ultrasound device. **Continuous monitoring** is usually offered if medical interventions such as an **epidural** or an **oxytocin** drip are being used, because of the extra stress that these may put on the baby. For more about the pros and cons of continuous monitoring see *www.aims.org.uk/information/ item/monitoring-your-babys-heartbeat-in-labour*

Early birth is a birth that is brought forward from the time at which spontaneous labour would have started, either by medical induction or a planned **caesarean**. In some cases, it is used to mean an induced or caesarean birth that takes place before full-term (40 weeks).

Early term birth is a birth that occurs after 37 full weeks of pregnancy but before the start of the 39th week. Though considered 'term' these babies are more likely to experience health problems including breathing difficulties than those born after the start of the 39th week.

Epidural (more accurately epidural analgesia) is a form of pain relief in which a fine needle is inserted into the space around the spinal cord and a tube is passed through this. The needle is taken out, and drugs are given through the tube to numb the nerves which carry messages about pain to the brain. The drugs are usually a mixture of a local anaesthetic and an opiate (morphine-like) drug. For more about the pros and cons of having an epidural see *www.aims.org.uk/information/ item/managing-labour#post-heading-9*

Expectant management is waiting for labour to start spontaneously rather than inducing it at a certain point in pregnancy.

Fetal compromise is diagnosed when there are signs of serious problems with a baby's well-being, such as reduced blood flow in the blood vessels of the placenta or concerns over the baby's heart rate.

(Fetal) Growth charts are used to check on how your baby is growing in the womb and to provide an estimate of what the birthweight will be. They may either record a midwife's regular measurements of how the 'bump' is growing or use ultrasound measurements of the baby's size.

Fetal Growth Restriction is the situation where a baby's normal growth is being affected by some problem, causing them to be smaller than expected. The causes of fetal growth restriction can include genetic problems, infection, or a problem with the working of the placenta. This is not the same as **SGA** as some small babies are growing as they should but are naturally small.

Forceps are a pair of metal instruments which look a bit like large spoons and can be fitted around a baby's head to enable a doctor to turn and/or pull the baby out. See also **Assisted birth**

GDG (Guideline Development Group) is a group of people responsible for drafting guidelines such as the NICE guidelines. In the case of NICE guidelines they will agree the review questions, consider the evidence and develop the recommendations. The GDG normally includes both healthcare and other professionals and user representatives.

Instrumental birth See **Assisted birth**

LGA (large-for-gestational-age) describes a baby who is at the upper end of the weight-range for that point in pregnancy. The usual definition is that a baby is LGA if they have an actual birthweight over 4000g (4kg or 8lb 13oz) or an estimated fetal weight which is in the top 90% of the population at that point in pregnancy. This means they are above the 90th centile on their **growth chart**.

Macrosomia/macrosomic – see **LGA**

Meta-analysis is a type of review of research evidence which combines the data from a number of **randomised controlled trials**. This can help to overcome the problem of such trials having too small a sample to detect a difference in rare outcomes, but the approach has limitations. For more on this see the AIMS Birth Information web page "Understanding Quantitative Research Evidence", *www.aims.org.uk/information/item/quantitative-research.*

Neonatal death is the death of baby within the first 28 days after birth. This is sometimes divided into early neonatal deaths which happen in the first week and late neonatal deaths which are between seven and 28 days after birth.

Ongoing pregnancies is an estimate of how many people were still pregnant at a certain week of pregnancy.

Oxytocin is a hormone which is produced in the brain during labour and stimulates the muscles of the womb to contract. It also has a positive effect on mood and promotes bonding between partners, parents and babies. A synthetic version of the same substance may be given through a drip into the hand or arm as a method of **augmentation** to try to start or strengthen contractions.

Perinatal deaths are the total deaths of babies beyond 24 weeks of pregnancy that occur before or during labour (**stillbirths**), plus those that occur shortly after birth (**neonatal deaths**). Usually this includes only neonatal deaths up to seven days after birth, but sometimes those occurring up to 28 days after birth (referred to as extended perinatal deaths).

Planned (elective) birth is one that is planned to take place at a certain point in pregnancy, either by induction or a planned caesarean.

Population studies (also known as observational studies) are studies that look at how outcomes differ between groups defined by one or more characteristics such as their age, or by a difference in the treatment that they receive. Mostly these are 'retrospective studies' which look back at the records of a population, often over a period of years. There are also 'prospective studies' which define the groups to be studied at the start of the research and then follow up what happens to people in these groups.

Pre-eclampsia is a usually mild but potential serious complication of pregnancy, which should be monitored closely, and may require a planned early birth (induction or caesarean). The main symptoms are high blood pressure and protein in the urine, which is why these are tested for at routine antenatal appointments.

Pre-term or premature birth is a birth which occurs before the end of the 37th week of pregnancy.

Prostaglandins are chemicals made by the body which have similar effects to hormones but are produced and act locally. There are many different types, including those that cause ripening of cervix in preparation for labour to begin. A version of these natural substances can be applied as a pessary as a way of inducing labour.

Induction of Labour

Randomised controlled trial (RCT) is a form of research study where people are randomly divided into two or more groups, each of which receives a different treatment, so that the outcomes can be compared. Ideally, such trials would be 'blinded', which means that neither the person in the trial, nor those caring for them know which group they are in. This is not usually possible in research about labour and birth.

Relative Risk is a measure of how much more common it is for a problem to occur in one group compared with another. For example, if a problem is observed twice as often in group B as in group A, then the relative risk for group B compared with group A would be 2.

SGA (small-for-gestational-age) describes a baby who is at the lower end of the weight-range for that point in pregnancy. The usual definition is that a baby is SGA if they have an actual birthweight or an estimated fetal weight which is in the lowest 10% of the population at that point in pregnancy. This means they are below the 10th centile on their **growth chart**. It is not the same as **fetal growth restriction**, as not all SGA babies are growing poorly in the womb – some are naturally small.

Statistically significant means that a result that is highly unlikely to have occurred by chance. Note that this is a technical use of the word 'significant'. It's not saying anything about the importance of the finding.

Stillbirth is the death of a baby that occurs after 24 weeks of pregnancy and before or during labour. Those that happen before labour starts are sometimes called 'antepartum stillbirths' and those that occur during labour as 'intrapartum stillbirths'. Those that occur before 24 weeks of pregnancy are referred to as miscarriages.

Term birth is a birth which occurs between the 37th and 42nd weeks of pregnancy.

Ventouse (see also **Assisted birth**) is a device with a plastic or metal cup which is placed on a baby's head and connected to a suction device. The suction creates a vacuum inside the cup so that it stays on the baby's head while the doctor or midwife pulls the baby out.

References

The links below were correct at the time of writing, but webpages are sometimes moved or changed. If a link appears to be broken, you should be able to find the page by typing the title into a search engine.

Acker D.B. *et al* "Risk factors for shoulder dystocia." Obstet. Gynecol. 66(6), 762–768 (1985). www.ncbi.nlm.nih.gov/pubmed/4069477

ACOG (The American College of Obstetricians and Gynecologists Committee on Obstetric Practice) "Definition of Term Pregnancy" Committee Opinion Number 579, November 2013 (Reaffirmed 2017) www.acog.org/Clinical-Guidance-and-Publications/Committee-Opinions/Committee-on-Obstetric-Practice/Definition-of-Term-Pregnancy

Alberico S. *et al* "Gestational diabetes and fetal growth acceleration: induction of labour versus expectant management." Minerva Ginecol. 2010 Dec;62(6):533-9. https://www.minervamedica.it/en/journals/minerva-ginecologica/article.php?cod=R09Y2010N06A0533

Alberico S. *et al* "Immediate delivery or expectant management in gestational diabetes at term: the ginexmal randomised controlled trial." BJOG: an international journal of obstetrics and gynaecology 2017;124(4):669-77. obgyn.onlinelibrary.wiley.com/doi/full/10.1111/1471-0528.14389

Alfirevic Z. et al Cochrane Review: Oxytocin for induction of labour (2009) www.cochrane.org/CD003246/PREG_oxytocin-for-induction-of-labour

Alfirevic Z. *et al* Cochrane review: "Continuous cardiotocography (CTG) as a form of electronic fetal monitoring (EFM) for fetal assessment during labour." 2017 www.cochranelibrary.com/cdsr/doi/10.1002/14651858.CD006066.pub3/full

Anim-Soumah M. *et al* Cochrane review: Epidural versus non-epidural or no analgesia for pain management in labour (2018) www.cochranelibrary.com/cdsr/doi/10.1002/14651858.CD000331.pub4/abstract

BarrettJ.F.R. *et al* "A Randomized Trial of Planned Cesarean or Vaginal Delivery for Twin Pregnancy" N Engl J Med 2013; 369:1295-1305 www.nejm.org/doi/full/10.1056/NEJMoa1214939

Bell A.F. *et al* Beyond labor: the role of natural and synthetic oxytocin in the transition to motherhood *J. Midwifery Womens Health. 59(1)*: 35–42. 2014 www.ncbi.nlm.nih.gov/pmc/articles/PMC3947469/

Biesty L.M. *et al* Cochrane Review "Planned birth at or near term for pregnant women with gestational diabetes and their infants" 2018 www.cochrane.org/CD012910/PREG_planned-birth-or-near-term-pregnant-women-gestational-diabetes-and-their-infants

Biesty L.M. *et al* Cochrane Review "Planned birth at or near term for improving health outcomes for pregnant women with pre-existing diabetes and their infants" 2018b www.cochranelibrary.com/cdsr/doi/10.1002/14651858.CD012948/full

Bingham J. *et al* "Recurrent shoulder dystocia: a review." Obstet. Gynecol. Surv. 65(3), 183–188 (2010). www.ncbi.nlm.nih.gov/pubmed/20214833

Birthplace in England Collaborative Group "Perinatal and maternal outcomes by planned place of birth for healthy women with low risk pregnancies: the Birthplace in England national prospective cohort study" BMJ 2011;343:d7400 www.bmj.com/content/343/bmj.d7400

Boers K.E. *et al* "Induction versus expectant monitoring for intrauterine growth restriction at term: randomised equivalence trial (DIGITAT)" BMJ 2010;341:c7087 www.bmj.com/content/341/bmj.c7087.long

Bohren M.A. *et al* Cochrane Review: "Continuous support for women during childbirth." (2017) www.cochranelibrary.com/cdsr/doi/10.1002/14651858.CD003766.pub6/full

Bond D.M. *et al* Cochrane review "Planned early delivery versus expectant management of the term suspected compromised baby for improving outcomes" (2015) www.cochranelibrary.com/cdsr/doi/10.1002/14651858.CD009433.pub2/full

Bond D.M. *et al* Cochrane review "Planned early birth versus expectant management for women with preterm prelabour rupture of membranes prior to 37 weeks' gestation for improving pregnancy outcome." (2017) www.cochranelibrary.com/cdsr/doi/10.1002/14651858.CD004735.pub4/full

Boulvain M. *et al* Cochrane review: "Membrane sweeping for induction of labour " (2005) www.cochrane.org/CD000451/PREG_membrane-sweeping-for-induction-of-labour

Boulvain M. *et al* Cochrane review "Induction of labour at or near term for suspected fetal macrosomia" (2016) www.cochranelibrary.com/cdsr/doi/10.1002/14651858.CD000938.pub2/full

Bricker L. & Lukas M. Cochrane review: "Amniotomy alone for induction of labour" (2000) www.cochrane.org/CD002862/PREG_amniotomy-alone-for-induction-of-labour

Broekhuijsen K. *et al* 2015 "Immediate delivery versus expectant monitoring for hypertensive disorders of pregnancy between 34 and 37 weeks of gestation (HYPITAT-II): an open-label, randomised controlled trial" The Lancet 385 (9986): 2492-2501 www.thelancet.com/journals/lancet/article/PIIS0140-6736(14)61998-X/fulltext

Buchanan S.L. *et al* "Trends and morbidity associated with oxytocin use in labour in nulliparas at term". Aust N Z J Obstet Gynaecol. 2012 Apr;52(2):173-8 www.ncbi.nlm.nih.gov/pubmed/22384940

Buckley S. "Undisturbed Birth" AIMS Journal, 2011, Vol 23 No 4 www.aims.org.uk/journal/item/undisturbed-birth

Bugg G.J. *et al* Cochrane review: "The effect/use of the drug oxytocin as a treatment for slow progress in labour" (2013) www.cochrane.org/CD007123/PREG_the-effectuse-of-the-drug-oxytocin-as-a-treatment-for-slow-progress-in-labour

Buhimschi *et al* "Rupture of the uterine scar during term labour: contractility or biochemistry?" BJOG 112: 38–42, 2004 obgyn.onlinelibrary.wiley.com/doi/pdf/10.1111/j.1471-0528.2004.00300.x

Cahill *et al*, 2007. Does a maximum dose of oxytocin affect risk for uterine rupture in candidates for vaginal birth after cesarean delivery? AJOG, Vol 197,5, November 2007, www.sciencedirect.com/science/article/abs/pii/S0002937807004929

Cahill *et al*, 2008. Higher maximum doses of oxytocin are associated with an unacceptably high risk for uterine rupture in patients attempting vaginal birth after cesarean delivery. AJOG, Volume 199, Issue 1, July 2008 www.sciencedirect.com/science/article/abs/pii/S0002937808002627

Carberry *et al* Cochrane review "Customised versus population-based growth charts as a screening tool for detecting small for gestational age infants in low-risk pregnant women" (2014) www.cochranelibrary.com/cdsr/doi/10.1002/14651858.CD008549.pub2/full

Cheong-See F. *et al* "Prospective risk of stillbirth and neonatal complications in twin pregnancies: systematic review and meta-analysis." BMJ. 2016;354:i4353. www.bmj.com/content/354/bmj.i4353

Chippington Derrick D. & Higson N. "Labour Induction at Term – How great is the risk of refusing it?" AIMS Journal 31 (1) 2019

Churchill D. Cochrane Review "Interventionist versus expectant care for severe pre-eclampsia before term" 2018 *et al* www.cochrane.org/CD003106/PREG_interventionist-versus-expectant-care-severe-pre-eclampsia-term

Coomarasamy A. *et al* "Accuracy of ultrasound biometry in the prediction of macrosomia: a systematic quantitative review." BJOG. 2005 Nov;112(11):1461-6. obgyn.onlinelibrary.wiley.com/doi/full/10.1111/j.1471-0528.2005.00702.x

Cotzias C.S. *et al* "Prospective risk of unexplained stillbirth in singleton pregnancies at term: population based analysis" BMJ. 1999 Jul 31; 319(7205): 287–288 www.ncbi.nlm.nih.gov/pmc/articles/PMC28178/

Davey M. and King J. "Caesarean section following induction of labour in uncomplicated first births- a population-based cross-sectional analysis of 42,950 births" BMC Pregnancy & Childbirth, April 2016, 16: 92 bmcpregnancychildbirth.biomedcentral.com/articles/10.1186/s12884-016-0869-0

Davies S. "Troubled Waters?" AIMS Journal, 2011, Vol 23 No 4 www.aims.org.uk/journal/item/troubled-waters

Dodd J.M. *et al* Cochrane review "Elective birth of women with an uncomplicated twin pregnancy from 37 weeks' gestation" 2014 www.cochrane.org/CD003582/ PREG_elective-birth-of-women-with-an-uncomplicated-twin-pregnancy-from-37-weeks-gestation

DoH National Framework for Diabetes 2001 www.gov.uk/government/publications/national-service-framework-diabetes

Downe S. *et al* Cochrane review "Routine vaginal examinations for assessing progress of labour to improve outcomes for women and babies at term" 2013 www.cochranelibrary.com/cdsr/doi/10.1002/14651858.CD010088.pub2/full

Dunn A.B. *et al* "The Maternal Infant Microbiome: Considerations for Labor and Birth" MCN Am J Matern Child Nurs. 2017 Nov-Dec; 42(6): 318–325. www.ncbi.nlm.nih.gov/pmc/articles/PMC5648605/

Egarter C.H.*et al* " Is induction of labor indicated in prolonged pregnancy? Results of a prospective randomised trial." Gynecologic and Obstetric Investigation 1989;27:6-9. www.karger.com/Article/Abstract/293605

Egarter C.H. *et al* " Uterine hyperstimulation after low-dose prostaglandin E2 therapy: Tocolytic treatment in 181 cases" *AJOG Volume 163, Issue 3*, Pages 794–796 (1990) www.ncbi.nlm.nih.gov/pubmed/1976296

Ek S. *et al* "Oligohydramnios in Uncomplicated Pregnancies beyond 40 Completed Weeks" Fetal Diagn Ther 2005;20:182–185 www.ncbi.nlm.nih.gov/pubmed/15824494

Enkin M. W. *et al* "A Guide to Effective Care in Pregnancy & Childbirth" Oxford University Press; 3rd edition, 2000

Fitzpatrick K.E. *et al* "Uterine rupture by intended mode of delivery in the UK: a national case-control study". PLoS Med 2012;9:e1001184. (The UKOSS study) journals.plos.org/plosmedicine/article?id=10.1371/journal.pmed.1001184

Friesen C.D. *et al* "Influence of Spontaneous or Induced Labor on Delivering the Macrosomic Fetus" Amer J Perinatol 1995; 12(1): 63-66 www.ncbi.nlm.nih.gov/pubmed/7710582

Fox H "Aging of the placenta" Archives of Disease in Childhood - Fetal and Neonatal Edition 1997;77:F171-F175 fn.bmj.com/content/fetalneonatal/77/3/F171.full.pdf

Gao L. *et al* "Steroid receptor coactivators 1 and 2 mediate fetal-to-maternal signaling that initiates parturition" *J Clin Invest. 125(7):*2808-24 2015 www.jci.org/articles/view/78544

Gardosi *et al* "Maternal and fetal risk factors for stillbirth: population based study" BMJ 2013; 346:f108 January 2013 www.bmj.com/content/346/bmj.f108

Geenes V. *et al* "Association of Severe Intrahepatic Cholestasis of Pregnancy with Adverse Pregnancy Outcomes: A Prospective Population-Based Case-Control Study" Hepatology. 2014 Apr; 59(4): 1482–1491. www.ncbi.nlm.nih.gov/pmc/articles/PMC4296226/

Glantz A. *et al* "Intrahepatic cholestasis of pregnancy: Relationships between bile acid levels and fetal complication rates." Hepatology. 2004 Aug;40(2):467-74. aasldpubs.onlinelibrary.wiley.com/doi/full/10.1002/hep.20336

Guise J.M. *et al* "Vaginal Birth After Cesarean: New Insights. Evidence Reports/Technology Assessments, No. 191"Agency for Healthcare Research and Quality; 2010. www.ncbi.nlm.nih.gov/books/NBK44571/

Gunn G.C. *et al* "Premature rupture of the fetal membranes" AJOG 106 (3): 469–483, 1970 www.ajog.org/article/0002-9378(70)90378-9/pdf

Hamza *et al* "Polyhydramnios: Causes, Diagnosis and Therapy" Geburtshilfe Frauenheilkd. 2013 Dec; 73(12): 1241–1246. www.ncbi.nlm.nih.gov/pmc/articles/PMC3964358/

Hamed H.O. *et al* "Pregnancy outcomes of expectant management of stable mild to moderate chronic hypertension as compared with planned delivery" International Journal of Obstetrics & Gynecology 127 (1): 15-10 2014 obgyn.onlinelibrary.wiley.com/doi/abs/10.1016/j.ijgo.2014.04.010

Hannah M.E. *et al* "Induction of labor as compared with serial antenatal monitoring in post-term pregnancy. A randomized controlled trial. The Canadian Multicenter Post-term Pregnancy Trial Group." N Engl J Med. 1992 Jun 11;326(24):1587-92 www.nejm.org/doi/10.1056/NEJM199206113262402?url_ver=Z39.88-2003&rfr_id=ori:rid:crossref.org&rfr_dat=cr_pub%3dwww.ncbi.nlm.nih.gov

Hannah M.E. *et al* "Induction of Labor Compared with Expectant Management for Prelabor Rupture of the Membranes at Term" N Engl J Med 1996; 334:1005-1010 www.nejm.org/doi/full/10.1056/NEJM199604183341601

Helmerhorst FM, Perquin DA, Donker D, Keirse MJ. Perinatal outcome of singletons and twins after assisted conception: a systematic review of controlled studies. BMJ 2004;328:261. www.ncbi.nlm.nih.gov/pmc/articles/PMC324454/#ref1

Henningsen A.A. *et al* "Risk of stillbirth and infant deaths after assisted reproductive technology: a Nordic study from the CoNARTaS† group" Human Reproduction, Volume 29, Issue 5, 1 May 2014, Pages 1090–1096 academic.oup.com/humrep/article/29/5/1090/674618

Hickey K. "Induction: First do no harm" AIMS Journal, 2019, Vol 31, No 1 www.aims.org.uk/journal/item/induction-care-bundles

Hodin S. The Lancet Maternal Health Series: "Beyond Too Little, Too Late and Too Much, Too Soon" 2016 www.mhtf.org/2016/10/17/the-lancet-maternal-health-series-beyond-too-little-too-late-and-too-much-too-soon/

Holman N. *et al* "Women with pre-gestational diabetes have a higher risk of stillbirth at all gestations after 32 weeks" Diabetic Medicine 31 (9) 2014 www.ncbi.nlm.nih.gov/pubmed/24836172

Howarth G.R. and Botha D.J. Cochrane review: "Amniotomy plus intravenous oxytocin for induction of labour" (2001) www.cochranelibrary.com/cdsr/doi/10.1002/14651858.CD003250/abstract

Jacquemyn Y. *et al* "Elective induction of labour increases caesarean section rate in low risk multiparous women" Journal of Obstetrics & Gynecology Volume 32 (3), 2012 www.tandfonline.com/doi/abs/10.3109/01443615.2011.645091?journalCode=ijog20

Jonsson M. "Induction of twin pregnancy and the risk of caesarean delivery: a cohort study" BMC Pregnancy and Childbirth 15:136 2015 bmcpregnancychildbirth.biomedcentral.com/articles/10.1186/s12884-015-0566-4

Jowitt M. "Should labour be induced for prolonged pregnancy?" Midwifery Matters 134, 2012 www.midwifery.org.uk/articles/midwifery-matters-autumn-2012-issue-134/

Jozwiak M. *et al* Cochrane review: Mechanical methods for induction of labour (2012) www.cochrane.org/CD001233/PREG_mechanical-methods-for-induction-of-labour

Jukic A.M. *et al* "Length of human pregnancy and contributors to its natural variation" Hum Reprod. 2013 Oct; 28(10): 2848–2855. www.ncbi.nlm.nih.gov/pmc/articles/PMC3777570/

Karkhanis P. and Patni S. "Polyhydramnios in singleton pregnancies: perinatal outcomes and management" The Obstetrician & Gynecologist 16:3 207-213 July 2014 obgyn.onlinelibrary.wiley.com/doi/10.1111/tog.12113

Katz V.L. and Bowes W.A. "Meconium aspiration syndrome: Reflections on a murky subject" AJOG January 1992 Volume 166, Issue 1, Part 1, Pages 171–183 www.ncbi.nlm.nih.gov/pubmed/1733193

Kavanagh J. *et al* Cochrane review "Breast stimulation for cervical ripening and induction of labour" (2005) www.cochranelibrary.com/cdsr/doi/10.1002/14651858.CD003392.pub2/full

Khambalia A.Z. *et al* "Predicting date of birth and examining the best time to date a pregnancy." Int J Gynaecol Obstet. 2013 Nov;123(2):105-9 www.ncbi.nlm.nih.gov/pubmed/23932061

Kjos S.L. *et al* "Insulin-requiring diabetes in pregnancy: a randomized trial of active induction of labor and expectant management" Am J Obstet Gynecol. 1993 Sep;169(3) www.ajog.org/article/0002-9378(93)90631-R/pdf

Knight H.E. *et al* "Perinatal mortality associated with induction of labour versus expectant management in nulliparous women aged 35 years or over: An English national cohort study" PLOS Medicine 2017 journals.plos.org/plosmedicine/article?id=10.1371/journal.pmed.1002425

Knight B. *et al* "Assessing the accuracy of ultrasound estimation of gestational age during routine antenatal care in in vitro fertilization (IVF) pregnancies" BMUS Volume: 26 (1): 49-53 2018. journals.sagepub.com/doi/full/10.1177/1742271X17751257

Koopmans C.M. *et al* "Induction of labour versus expectant monitoring for gestational hypertension or mild pre-eclampsia after 36 weeks' gestation (HYPITAT): a multicentre, open-label randomised controlled trial." Lancet. 2009 Sep 19;374(9694):979-988 www.thelancet.com/journals/lancet/article/PIIS0140-6736(09)60736-4/fulltext

Kroll-Desrosiers A.R. *et al* "Association of peripartum synthetic oxytocin administration and depressive and anxiety disorders within the first postpartum year" Depress. Anxiety 2017; 34(2): 137-146 onlinelibrary.wiley.com/doi/full/10.1002/da.22599

Landon M.B. *et al* "Maternal and perinatal outcomes associated with a trial of labor after prior cesarean delivery". N Engl J Med 2004;351:2581–9. www.nejm.org/doi/10.1056/NEJMoa040405?url_ver=Z39.88-2003&rfr_id=ori:rid:crossref.org&rfr_dat=cr_pub%3dwww.ncbi.nlm.nih.gov

Lawrence A. *et al* Cochrane Review: "Maternal positions and mobility during first stage labour." (2013) www.cochranelibrary.com/cdsr/doi/10.1002/14651858.CD003934.pub4/full

Leeman L. and Almond D. "Isolated oligohydramnios at term: Is induction indicated?" 54: 1 · The Journal of Family Practice 2005 www.mdedge.com/familymedicine/article/60309/womens-health/isolated-oligohydramnios-term-induction-indicated

Lie R.T. *et al* "Maternal and paternal influences on length of pregnancy. "Obstetrics & Gynecology. 107(4):880-885, APR 2006" journals.lww.com/greenjournal/fulltext/2006/04000/Maternal_and_Paternal_Influences_on_Length_of.22.aspx

Lurie S. *et al* "Induction of labor at 38 to 39 weeks of gestation reduces the incidence of shoulder dystocia in gestational diabetic patients class A2" Am J Perinatol. 1996 Jul;13(5):293-6. www.ncbi.nlm.nih.gov/pubmed/8863948

Magann E.F. *et al* "Amniotic Fluid and the Clinical Relevance of the Sonographically Estimated Amniotic Fluid Volume" Journal of Ultrasound Medicine 30:11, 1573-1585 November 2011 onlinelibrary.wiley.com/doi/full/10.7863/jum.2011.30.11.1573?sid=nlm%3Apubmed

Maiti K. *et al* "Evidence that fetal death is associated with placental aging." Am J Obstet Gynecol. 2017 Oct;217(4):441.2017 www.ajog.org/article/S0002-9378(17)30756-1/fulltext

Mandruzzato G. *et al* "Guidelines for the management of postterm pregnancy." J Perinat Med. 2010 Mar;38(2):111-9 www.ncbi.nlm.nih.gov/pubmed/20156009/

Martis R. *et al* Cochrane Review "Treatments to improve pregnancy outcomes for women who develop diabetes during pregnancy: an overview of Cochrane systematic reviews" www.cochrane.org/CD012327/PREG_treatments-improve-pregnancy-outcomes-women-who-develop-diabetes-during-pregnancy-overview-cochrane

MBRRACE "Perinatal Mortality Surveillance Report for 2015 Births" published June 2017 www.npeu.ox.ac.uk/mbrrace-uk/reports/perinatal-mortality-surveillance

MBRRACE "Saving Lives, Improving Mothers' Care" published November 2018 www.npeu.ox.ac.uk/downloads/files/mbrrace-uk/reports/MBRRACE-UK%20Maternal%20Report%202018%20-%20Web%20Version.pdf

Mei-Dan E. *et al* "The effect of induction method in twin pregnancies: a secondary analysis for the twin birth study" BMC Pregnancy Childbirth. 2017; 17: 9 bmcpregnancychildbirth.biomedcentral.com/articles/10.1186/s12884-016-1201-8

Menticoglu S.M. and Hall S.F. "Routine induction of labour at 41 weeks: nonsensus consensus" BJOG 109 (5) May 2002 pp485-491 obgyn.onlinelibrary.wiley.com/doi/abs/10.1111/j.1471-0528.2002.01004.x

Menticoglou S. "Shoulder dystocia: incidence, mechanisms, and management strategies" Int J Womens Health. 2018; 10: 723–732. www.ncbi.nlm.nih.gov/pmc/articles/PMC6233701/

Middleton P. *et al* Cochrane Review: "Planned early birth versus expectant management (waiting) for prelabour rupture of membranes at term (37 weeks or more)" (2017) www.cochranelibrary.com/cdsr/doi/10.1002/14651858.CD005302.pub3/full

Middleton P. *et al* Cochrane review: "Induction of labour in women with normal pregnancies at or beyond term" (2018) www.cochrane.org/CD004945/PREG_induction-labour-women-normal-pregnancies-or-beyond-term

Mogren I. *et al* "Recurrence of prolonged pregnancy." International Journal of Epidemiology, Volume 28, Issue 2, 1 April 1999, Pages 253–257 academic.oup.com/ije/article/28/2/253/655234

Morken N-H *et al* "Perinatal mortality by gestational week and size at birth in singleton pregnancies at and beyond term: a nationwide population-based cohort study" BMC Pregnancy and Childbirth 2014 14:172 bmcpregnancychildbirth.biomedcentral.com/articles/10.1186/1471-2393-14-172

Mozurkewich E.L.*et al* "Methods of induction of labour: a systematic review" BMC Pregnancy and Childbirth 11:84 (2011) bmcpregnancychildbirth.biomedcentral. com/articles/10.1186/1471-2393-11-84

Muglu J. *et al* "Risks of stillbirth and neonatal death with advancing gestation at term: A systematic review and meta-analysis of cohort studies of 15 million pregnancies." Nabhan A.F. and Abdelmoula Y.A. Cochrane review "Amniotic fluid index versus single deepest vertical pocket as a screening test for preventing adverse pregnancy outcome" 2008 www.cochranelibrary.com/cdsr/doi/10.1002/14651858. CD006593.pub2/media/CDSR/CD006593/CD006593.pdf

NHS Maternity Statistics, 2017-18 digital.nhs.uk/pubs/maternity1718

Nesbitt TS *et al* "Shoulder dystocia and associated risk factors with macrosomic infants born in California." Am. J. Obstet. Gynecol. 179(2), 476–480 (1998) www. ajog.org/article/S0002-9378(98)70382-5/fulltext

NICE Clinical Guideline: Inducing Labour (2008) www.nice.org.uk/guidance/ cg70

NICE Clinical Guideline: Caesarean Section (2011) www.nice.org.uk/guidance/ cg132

NICE Clinical Guideline: Intrapartum care for healthy women and babies (2014, updated 2017) www.nice.org.uk/guidance/cg190

NICE Interventional Procedures Guideline: Insertion of a double balloon catheter for induction of labour in pregnant women without previous caesarean section (2015) www.nice.org.uk/guidance/ipg528

NICE Clinical Guideline: Diabetes in pregnancy: management from preconception to the postnatal period (2015b) www.nice.org.uk/guidance/ng3

NICE Clinical Guideline: Hypertension in Pregnancy (2019) www.nice.org.uk/ guidance/ng133

NICE Clinical Guideline: Intrapartum care for women with existing medical conditions or obstetric complications and their babies (2019b) www.nice.org.uk/ guidance/ng121

NICE Clinical Guideline: Twin and Triplet pregnancies (2019c) www.nice.org.uk/ guidance/cg129

Oberg A.S. *et al* "Maternal and Fetal Genetic Contributions to Postterm Birth: Familial Clustering in a Population-Based Sample of 475,429 Swedish Births" American Journal of Epidemiology, Volume 177, Issue 6, 15 March 2013, Pages 531–537 academic.oup.com/aje/article/177/6/531/160108

Office for National Statistics "Birth Characteristics, England and Wales: 2017" published January 2019 www.ons.gov.uk/ peoplepopulationandcommunity/birthsdeathsandmarriages/livebirths/bulletins/ birthcharacteristicsinenglandandwales/2017

Ovadia C. *et al* "Association of adverse perinatal outcomes of intrahepatic cholestasis of pregnancy with biochemical markers: results of aggregate and individual patient data meta-analyses." The Lancet 2019; DOI: dx.doi. org/10.1016/S0140-6736(18)31877-4

Patel R.R. *et al* "Does gestation vary by ethnic group? A London-based study of over 122,000 pregnancies with spontaneous onset of labour." Int J Epidemiol. 2004 Feb;33(1):107-13. academic.oup.com/ije/article/33/1/107/668109

Putnam K. *et al* Randomized clinical trial evaluating the frequency of membrane sweeping with an unfavorable cervix at 39 weeks *Int J Womens Health. 2011; 3*: 287–294 www.ncbi.nlm.nih.gov/pmc/articles/PMC3163659/

Qin J *et al* "Assisted reproductive technology and the risk of pregnancy-related complications and adverse pregnancy outcomes in singleton pregnancies: a meta-analysis of cohort studies" Fertility and Sterility 105, 1, January 2016, Pages 73-85. e6 www.ncbi.nlm.nih.gov/pubmed/26453266

Roberts A. "Informed Decision Making – does research help us?" AIMS Journal, 2019, Vol 31, No 1 www.aims.org.uk/journal/item/35-39

RCOG 2001 "Induction of Labour" (Evidence based clinical guideline no. 9)

RCOG 2011 "Cardiac Disease and Pregnancy" (Good Practice No.13) www.rcog.org. uk/globalassets/documents/guidelines/goodpractice13cardiacdiseaseandpregnancy. pdf

RCOG 2011b "Obstetric Cholestasis" Green–top Guideline No. 43 www.rcog.org. uk/globalassets/documents/guidelines/gtg_43.pdf

RCOG 2012 "In Vitro Fertilisation: Perinatal Risks and Early Childhood Outcomes" (Scientific Impact Paper No. 8) www.rcog.org.uk/globalassets/ documents/guidelines/scientific-impact-papers/sip_8.pdf

RCOG 2012b Green-top Guide "Shoulder Dystocia" www.rcog.org.uk/en/ guidelines-research-services/guidelines/gtg42/

RCOG 2013 "Induction of Labour at Term in Older Mothers" (Scientific Impact Paper No. 34) www.rcog.org.uk/en/guidelines-research-services/guidelines/sip34/

RCOG 2013b Query Bank Labour induction after IVF Published: 20/05/2013

RCOG 2013c "Small-for-Gestational-Age Fetus, Investigation and Management" (Green-top Guideline No. 31) www.rcog.org.uk/en/guidelines-research-services/ guidelines/gtg31/

RCOG 2015 "Greentop Guide 45 Birth After Previous Caesarean" https://www. rcog.org.uk/en/guidelines-research-services/guidelines/gtg45/

RCOG 2015b "Obtaining Valid Consent" (Clinical Governance Advice No. 6) www.rcog.org.uk/en/guidelines-research-services/guidelines/clinical-governance-advice-6/

RCOG 2015c Patient Information Leaflet "Umbilical cord prolapse in late pregnancy"

RCOG 2017 "Prevention of Early-onset Neonatal Group B Streptococcal Disease" (Greentop Guide number 36) obgyn.onlinelibrary.wiley.com/doi/full/10.1111/1471-0528.14821

RCOG 2019 "Care of Women Presenting with Suspected Preterm Prelabour Rupture of Membranes from 24+0 Weeks of Gestation (Green-top Guideline No. 73)obgyn.onlinelibrary.wiley.com/doi/10.1111/1471-0528.15803

Reddy U.M. *et al* "Maternal age and the risk of stillbirth throughout pregnancy in the United States." Am J Obstet Gynecol. 2006 Sep;195(3):764-70. www.ajog.org/article/S0002-9378(06)00743-5/fulltext

Rosenstein M.G. *et al* "The risk of stillbirth and infant death stratified by gestational age in women with gestational diabetes." Am J Obstet Gynecol Apr 2012, 206 (4) 309 www.ncbi.nlm.nih.gov/pmc/articles/PMC3403365/

Sanchez-Ramos L. *et al* "Expectant management versus labor induction for suspected fetal macrosomia: a systematic review." Obstet Gynecol. 2002 Nov;100(5 Pt 1):997-1002 www.ncbi.nlm.nih.gov/pubmed/12423867

Sanchez-Ramos L, Olivier F, Delke I, Kaunitz AM. Labor induction versus expectant management for postterm pregnancies: a systematic review with meta-analysis. Obstet Gynecol. 2003;101:1312–8. www.ncbi.nlm.nih.gov/pubmed/12798542

Savitz D.A. *et al* "Influence of gestational age on the time from spontaneous rupture of the chorioamniotic membranes to the onset of labor." Am J Perinatol. 1997 Mar;14(3):129-33. www.thieme-connect.com/products/ejournals/abstract/10.1055/s-2007-994112

Seaward P.G. *et al* "International Multicentre Term Prelabor Rupture of Membranes Study: evaluation of predictors of clinical chorioamnionitis and postpartum fever in patients with prelabor rupture of membranes at term" *Am J Obstet Gynecol 177(5):*1024-9 (1997) www.ncbi.nlm.nih.gov/pubmed/9396886

Seaward P.G. *et al* "International multicenter term PROM study: evaluation of predictors of neonatal infection in infants born to patients with premature rupture of membranes at term. Premature Rupture of the Membranes." *Am J Obstet Gynecol 179(3 Pt 1):*635-9 (1998) www.ncbi.nlm.nih.gov/pubmed/9757963

Seijmonsbergen-Schermers A.E. *et al* "Which level of risk justifies routine induction of labor for healthy women?" *Sexual and Reproductive Health, in press November 2019* www.sciencedirect.com/science/article/abs/pii/S1877575619302332

Sherer D.M. & Langer O. "Oligohydramnios: use and misuse in clinical management" Editorial in Ultrasound Obstet Gynecol 2001; 18: 411–419 obgyn.onlinelibrary.wiley.com/doi/pdf/10.1046/j.1469-0705.2001.00570.x

Shrem G. *et al* "Isolated Oligohydramnios at Term as an Indication for Labor Induction: A Systematic Review and Meta-Analysis." Fetal Diagn Ther. 2016;40(3):161-173. www.karger.com/Article/FullText/445948

Simpson M. *et al* "Raspberry leaf in pregnancy: its safety and efficacy in labor." J Midwifery Womens Health. 2001 Mar-Apr;46(2):51-9. www.ncbi.nlm.nih.gov/pubmed/11370690

Smith C.A. *et al* Cochrane Review: "Acupuncture and Acupressure for Induction of Labour" (2017) www.cochrane.org/CD002962/PREG_acupuncture-or-acupressure-induction-labour

Smith C.V. *et al* "Relation of mild idiopathic polyhydramnios to perinatal outcome." Obstet Gynecol. 1992 Mar;79(3):387-9. www.ncbi.nlm.nih.gov/pubmed/1738520

Smith G.C.S. "Use of time to event analysis to estimate the normal duration of human pregnancy" Human Reproduction, Volume 16, Issue 7, 1 July 2001, Pages 1497–1500 academic.oup.com/humrep/article/16/7/1497/693431

Smyth R.M.D. *et al* Cochrane review "Amniotomy for shortening spontaneous labour" (2013) www.cochrane.org/CD006167/PREG_amniotomy-for-shortening-spontaneous-labour

Taipale P. and Hiilesmaa V. "Predicting delivery date by ultrasound and last menstrual period in early gestation." Obstet Gynecol. 2001 Feb;97(2):189-94. www.ncbi.nlm.nih.gov/pubmed/11165580

Tajik P. *et al* "Using vaginal Group B Streptococcus colonisation in women with preterm premature rupture of membranes to guide the decision for immediate delivery: a secondary analysis of the PPROMEXIL trials." BJOG 2014 Sep;121(10):1263-72 obgyn.onlinelibrary.wiley.com/doi/full/10.1111/1471-0528.12889

Tan P.C. *et al* "Effect of Coitus at Term on Length of Gestation, Induction of Labor, and Mode of Delivery" Obstetrics & Gynecology. 108(1):134-140 (2006) www.ncbi.nlm.nih.gov/pubmed/16816067

Thomas J. *et al* Cochrane Review: Vaginal prostaglandin (PGE2 and PGF2a) for induction of labour at term (2014) www.cochrane.org/CD003101/PREG_vaginal-prostaglandin-pge2-and-pgf2a-for-induction-of-labour-at-term

Ulmsten U. *et al* "Intracervical vs intravaginal PGE2 for induction of labor at term in patients with an unfavorable cervix." Archives of Gynecology 1985;236:243-8. link.springer.com/article/10.1007%2FBF02133942

Unsworth J. and Vause S. "Meconium in labour" Obstetrics, Gynecology & Reproductive Medicine October 2010 Volume 20, Issue 10, Pages 289–294 www.obstetrics-gynaecology-journal.com/article/S1751-7214(10)00112-0/abstract

Vardo J.H. *et al* "Maternal and neonatal morbidity among nulliparous women undergoing elective induction of labor." J. Reprod. Med. 2011 Jan-Feb;56(1-2):25-30. www.ncbi.nlm.nih.gov/pubmed/21366123

Vrouenraets F.P. *et al* "Bishop score and risk of cesarean delivery after induction of labor in nulliparous women" Obstet. Gynecol. 2005 Apr;105(4):690-7 www.ncbi. nlm.nih.gov/pubmed/15802392

Walker K.F. *et al* "Randomized Trial of Labor Induction in Women 35 Years of Age or Older" (The "35/39 trial") N Engl J Med 2016; 374:813-822 2016 www.nejm. org/doi/full/10.1056/NEJMoa1509117

Weeks J.W. *et al* "Fetal macrosomia: Does antenatal prediction affect delivery route and birth outcome?" AJOG Volume 173, Issue 4, Pages 1215–1219 1995 www. ajog.org/article/0002-9378(95)91356-4/abstract

Wennerholm U.B. *et al* "Induction of labor versus expectant management for post-date pregnancy: is there sufficient evidence for a change in clinical practice?" Acta Obstet Gynecol. 2009;88:6–17 www.ncbi.nlm.nih.gov/pubmed/19140042

Whitworth M. *et al* Cochrane Review: "Routine compared with selective ultrasound in early pregnancy" (2015) www.cochrane.org/CD007058/PREG_ routine-compared-selective-ultrasound-early-pregnancy

Wickham S. "The War on Group B Strep" AIMS Journal 2003, Vol 15, No 4 www. aims.org.uk/journal/item/the-war-on-group-b-strep

Widdows K. *et al* "Evaluation of the implementation of the Saving Babies' Lives Care Bundle in early adopter NHS Trusts in England. Maternal and Fetal Health Research Centre, University of Manchester, Manchester, UK. 2018. www. manchester.ac.uk/discover/news/action-plan-can-prevent-over-600-stillbirths-a-year/

Wojcieszek A.M. *et al* Cochrane Review "Antibiotics for prelabour rupture of membranes at or near term" (2014) www.cochranelibrary.com/cdsr/ doi/10.1002/14651858.CD001807.pub2/full

Yancey M.K. *et al* "The accuracy of late antenatal screening cultures in predicting genital group B streptococcal colonization at delivery." Obstet Gynecol. 1996 Nov;88(5):811-5 www.ncbi.nlm.nih.gov/pubmed/8885919/

Zhang G. *et al* "Genetic Associations with Gestational Duration and Spontaneous Preterm Birth." N Engl J Med 2017; 377:1156-1167 www.nejm.org/doi/ full/10.1056/NEJMoa1612665?query=featured_home

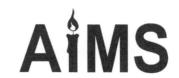

AIMS

There for your mother

Here for you

Help us to be there for your daughters

www.aims.org.uk

Twitter – @AIMS_online

Facebook – www.facebook.com/AIMSUK

Helpline

helpline@aims.org.uk

0300 365 0663